The Juice Lady's
LIVING FOODS
Revolution

Cherie Calbom

SILOAM

Most CHARISMA HOUSE BOOK GROUP products are available at special quantity discounts for bulk purchase for sales promotions, premiums, fund-raising, and educational needs. For details, write Charisma House Book Group, 600 Rinehart Road, Lake Mary, Florida 32746, or telephone (407) 333-0600.

THE JUICE LADY'S LIVING FOODS REVOLUTION by Cherie Calbom
Published by Siloam
Charisma Media/Charisma House Book Group
600 Rinehart Road, Lake Mary, Florida 32746
www.charismahouse.com

Visit the author's website at www.cheriecalbom.com.

Library of Congress Cataloging-in-Publication Data
Calbom, Cherie.
    The juice lady's living foods revolution : eat your way to health, detoxification, and weight loss with delicious juices and raw / Cherie Calbom.
    Summary: "Nutrition expert Cherie Calbom explains the benefits of raw foods, based on new scientific research that shows that biophotons in plants carry light energy into our bodies, which helps our cells communicate with each other"-- Provided by publisher.
    Includes bibliographical references and index.
    ISBN 978-1-61638-363-3 (pbk.) -- ISBN 978-1-61638-431-9 (e-book) 1. Raw food diet. I. Title.
    RM237.5.C275 2011
    613.2'6--dc22
                                      2011011388

This book contains the opinions and ideas of its author. It is solely for informational and educational purposes and should not be regarded as a substitute for professional medical treatment. The nature of your body's health condition is complex and unique. Therefore, you should consult a health professional before you begin any new exercise, nutrition, or supplementation program or if you have questions about your health. Neither the author nor the publisher shall be liable or responsible for any loss or damage allegedly arising from any information or suggestion in this book.

The statements in this book about consumable products or food have not been evaluated by the Food and Drug Administration. The recipes in this book are to be followed exactly as written. The publisher is not responsible for your specific health or allergy needs that may require medical supervision. The publisher is not responsible for any adverse reactions to the consumption of food or products that have been suggested in this book.

While the author has made every effort to provide accurate telephone numbers and Internet addresses at the time of publication, neither the publisher nor the author assumes any responsibility for errors or for changes that occur after publication.

13 14 15 16 17 — 9 8 7 6 5 4 3 2
Printed in Canada

To Abba, the Source of all light and life

Acknowledgments

To those who have assisted me with this book, I am truly grateful.

- To my editor, Debbie Marrie: You're the best! You've added such valuable input to this book. Your dedication to excellence has amazed me. I'm truly honored to have you as my editor.

- I also wish to express my deep and lasting appreciation to all the other people who have helped to make *The Juice Lady's Living Foods Revolution* a success.

- I want to thank Trillium (the original Juiceman juicer company) and the founders Steve and Rick Cesari for choosing me as your "Juice Lady" in 1990. I offer my heartfelt gratitude for believing in me when I was still a student at Bastyr University. This set a course for my life that has been the greatest adventure I could ever have hoped for in helping people find health and the vitality to fulfill their purpose.

- I want to thank my husband of twenty-six years, Fr. John, for the love and support you have given me all these years. You believed in me when I didn't even believe in myself. You helped me find my life's path as a nutritionist through your Living on Purpose classes. And you've cheered me on with each step of my journey, endless hours of writing, where you've had to take a backseat from time to time to my writing projects, and "go it alone" occasionally. Thank you, my buddy, from the bottom of my heart.

- Lastly, I want to thank the Holy Trinity and the angels who have assisted me in writing this book. To my dear heavenly Father, Jesus Christ, and Holy Spirit, thank You for guiding me throughout this project. You showed me Your ways of wisdom, creativity, and truth as to how to care for the human body. You've guided me to the fountain of life in the juicing and cleansing programs I've been able to develop. Thank You for the health I've come to enjoy. I also thank You for the awesome responsibility of helping other people discover a way of life that truly promotes health. For the blessings You have given me and Your unconditional love, I am so very grateful.

Contents

Foreword

IN THE BIBLE, our bodies are called the temple of God. Since I was diagnosed with an incurable illness seventeen years ago, I have chosen to take great care of my temple by consuming only the healthiest foods and beverages. As a husband and father of three young children, caring for my family's health is a top priority. To maintain extraordinary health, I start each morning with fresh green vegetable juice. In fact, raw living foods have become the cornerstone of my daily diet. Raw, living foods are loaded with vitamins, minerals, antioxidants—and most importantly, enzymes. Enzymes are bioactive proteins that are responsible for virtually all of the major and minor functions of the body. Food and digestive enzymes help to breakdown the proteins, carbohydrates, fats, and dairy we consume in our meals.

Since I firmly believe that you're not what you eat but what you digest, I highly recommend reading and following the principles found in Cherie Calbom's new book, *The Juice Lady's Living Foods Revolution*. In this highly engaging book, you'll learn which foods and beverages will supply you with the building blocks for good health. With great information and delicious, healthy recipes, *The Juice Lady's Living Foods Revolution* is a guide to healthy eating no family should be without. Whether you're looking for the most nutritious appetizers, entrees, beverages, snacks, or desserts, *The Juice Lady's Living Foods Revolution* will deliver.

—JORDAN RUBIN
FOUNDER AND CEO, GARDEN OF LIFE
NEW YORK TIMES BEST-SELLING AUTHOR OF *THE MAKER'S DIET*

Raw Foods Are Living Foods

If you haven't got your health, then you haven't got anything.
—Count Rugen, *The Princess Bride* (1987)

MANY PEOPLE ARE turning to raw foods as a lifestyle for weight loss and health improvements. Consumption of living foods is becoming popular with mainstream Americans as well as celebrities. Demi Moore, Carol Alt, Uma Thurman, Alicia Silverstone, Donna Karan, Lisa Bonet, Robin Williams, Woody Harrelson, Natalie Portman, Sting, Beyoncé, Jason Mraz, Madonna, Cher, Pierce Brosnan, Daryl Hannah, Susan Sarandon, Margaret Cho, Angela Bassett, Edward Norton, Brooke Burke, David Duchovny, and Tea Leoni have all publicly embraced or praised raw food, and some are full-time raw foodists. When interviewed, they have publicly stated that a raw food diet helps them lose weight or gain numerous other benefits such as a greater sense of well-being, clearer thinking, fewer illnesses, clearer skin, more energy, and less need for medication.

Celebrity chefs like Charlie Trotter, who offers raw dishes in his Chicago restaurant, have helped to place living foods in the headlines. Stars and average people like you and me—from New York to San Francisco—can be found dining at living food restaurants these days. Recently I gave a raw food lecture at Café Gratitude in San Rafael. There are six Café Gratitude restaurants in the greater San Francisco Bay Area. I was surprised that on a weeknight the restaurant was filled with a wide variety of folks. Move down the California coast to the Hollywood area, and you'll find at least seven live food restaurants where you just might find a star or two sipping a fresh juice and eating a raw pizza or enchilada. In Seattle, you can enjoy raw cuisine at three raw restaurants. I discovered gourmet entrees at Daily Juice in Austin, Texas. And if you're in Manhattan, there's at least a half dozen choices to delight your palate.

Recently, a reader of my book *The Juice Lady's Turbo Diet* wrote, "Could this finally be the solution to my health problems? I think I have a lot of relearning to do. A bit overwhelming, but I am determined. Let the journey begin!"

It's time for your journey to begin. *The Juice Lady's Living Foods Revolution* can change your life just as it has changed the lives of thousands of people who have adopted this plan for themselves—and just as it changed mine. That's why I wrote this book—to help you find the healing, vitality-producing power of living foods. You don't have to become an all-raw foodist. I'm not. I am encouraging you to get more raw food in your diet and to make it a bit more than half of the food you eat every day. Juicing and green smoothies represent one way to help you reach that goal quickly and easily.

My life changed years ago when I discovered the healing power of freshly made juice and raw and whole foods. I'd like to share my story with you.

I Wondered If I Would I Ever Be Well Again

I sat by the window in my father's home staring at the snow-topped mountains in the distance, imagining that people were enjoying the hiking trails and perhaps someone was climbing the mountain that day. It was early June, and the weather was beautiful. I wished I had the strength to just walk around the block. But I was too sick and tired—I could barely walk around the house. I had been sick for a couple of years and just kept getting worse. "Will I ever be well again?" I wondered.

When I turned thirty, I had to quit my job. I had chronic fatigue syndrome and fibromyalgia that made me so sick I couldn't work. I felt as though I had a never-ending flu. Constantly feverish with swollen glands and perennially lethargic, I was also in constant pain. My body ached as though I'd been bounced around in a washing machine.

I had moved back to my father's home in Colorado to try and recover. But not one doctor had an answer as to what I should do to facilitate healing. So I went to some health food stores and browsed around, talked with employees, and read a few books. I decided that everything I'd been doing—like eating fast food, granola for dinner, and not eating vegetables—was tearing down my health rather than healing my body. I read about juicing and whole foods, and it made sense. So I bought a juicer and designed a program I could follow.

I juiced and ate a nearly perfect diet of live and whole foods for three months. There were ups and downs throughout. I had days where I felt encouraged that I was making some progress but other days where I felt worse. Those were discouraging and made me wonder if health was the elusive dream. No one told me about detox reactions, which was what I was experiencing. I was obviously very toxic, and my body was cleansing away all that stuff that had made me sick. This caused some not-so-good days amid the promising ones.

But one morning I woke up early—early for me, which was around 8:00 a.m.—without an alarm sounding off. I felt like someone had given me a new body in the night. I had so much energy I actually wanted to go jogging. What had happened? This new sensation of health had just appeared with the morning sun. But actually my body had been healing all along; it just had not manifested until that day. What a wonderful sense of being alive! I looked and felt completely renewed.

With my juicer in tow and a new lifestyle fully embraced, I returned to Southern California a couple weeks later to finish writing my first book. For nearly a year it was "ten steps forward" with great health and more energy and stamina than I'd ever remembered.

Then, all of a sudden, I took a giant step back.

The Event That Took My Breath Away

July fourth was a beautiful day like so many others in Southern California. I celebrated the holiday with friends that evening at a backyard barbecue. We put on jackets to insulate against the cool evening air and watched fireworks light up the night sky. I returned just before midnight to the house I was sitting for vacationing friends who lived in a lovely neighborhood not far from some family members. I was in bed just a bit after midnight.

I woke up shivering some time later. "Why is it so cold?" I wondered as I rolled over to see the clock; it was 3:00 a.m. That's when I noticed that the door was open to the backyard. "Wonder how that happened?" I thought as I was about to get up to close and lock it. That's when I noticed him crouched in the shadows of the corner of the room—a shirtless young guy in shorts. I blinked twice, trying to deny what I was seeing.

Instead of running, he leaped off the floor and ran toward me. He pulled a pipe from his shorts and began attacking me, beating me repeatedly over the head and yelling, "Now you are dead!" We fought, or I should say I tried to defend myself and grab the pipe. It finally flew out of his hands. That's when he choked me to unconsciousness. I felt life leaving my body. In those last few seconds, I knew I was dying. "This is it, the end of my life," I thought. I felt sad for the people who loved me and how they would feel about this tragic event. Then I felt my spirit leave in a sensation of popping out of my body and floating upward. Suddenly everything was peaceful and still. I sensed I was traveling, at what seemed like the speed of light, through black space. I saw what looked like lights twinkling in the distance.

But all of a sudden I was back in my body, outside the house, clinging to a fence at the end of the dog run. I don't know how I got there. I screamed for help with all the breath I had. It was my third scream that took all my strength. I felt it would be my last. Each time I screamed, I passed out and landed on the cement. I then had to pull myself up again. But this time, a neighbor heard me and sent her husband to help. Within a short time I was on my way to the hospital.

Lying on a cold gurney at 4:30 a.m. chilled to the bone, in and out of consciousness, I tried to assess my injuries, which was virtually impossible. When I finally looked at my right hand, I almost passed out again. My ring finger was barely hanging on by a small piece of skin. My hand was split open, and I could see deep inside. The next thing I knew, I was being wheeled off to surgery. Later I learned that I had suffered serious injuries to my head, neck, back, and right hand, with multiple head wounds and part of my scalp torn from my head. I also incurred numerous cracked teeth that resulted in several root canals and crowns months later.

My right hand sustained the most severe injuries, with two knuckles crushed to mere bone fragments that had to be held together by three metal pins. Six months after the attack I still couldn't use it. The cast I wore—with bands holding up the ring finger, which had almost been torn from my hand, and various odd-shaped molded parts—looked like something from a science-fiction movie. I felt and looked worse than hopeless, with a shaved top of my head, totally red and swollen eyes, a gash on my face, a useless right hand, terrorizing fear, and barely enough energy to get dressed in the morning.

I was an emotional wreck. I couldn't sleep at night—not even a minute. It was torturous. Never mind that I was staying with a cousin and his family. There was no need to worry about safety from a practical point of view, but that made no difference emotionally. I'd lie in bed all night and stare at the ceiling or the bedroom door. I had five lights that I kept on all night. I'd try to read, but my eyes would sting. I could sleep for only a little while during the day.

But the worst part was the pain in my soul that nearly took my breath away. All the emotional pain of the attack joined up with the pain and trauma of my past for an emotional tsunami. My past had been riddled with loss, trauma, and anxiety. My brother died when I was two. My mother had died of cancer when I was six. I couldn't remember much about her death—the memories seemed blocked. But my cousin said I fainted at her funeral. That told me the impact was huge.

I lived for the next three years with my maternal grandparents and father. But Grandpa John, the love of my life, died when I was nine—the loss was immeasurable. Four years later my father was involved in a very tragic situation that would take far too long to discuss here, but to sum it up—it was horrific. He was no longer in my daily life. I felt terrified about my future. My grandmother was eighty-six. I had no idea how many more years she would live. The next year I moved to Oregon to live with an aunt and uncle until I graduated from high school.

As you can probably imagine, wrapped in my soul was a huge amount of anguish and pain. It took every ounce of my will, faith and trust in God, deep spiritual work, alternative medical help, extra vitamins and minerals, vegetable juicing, emotional release, healing prayer, and numerous detox programs to heal physically, mentally, and emotionally. I met a nutritionally minded physician who had healed his own slow mending broken bones with lots of vitamin-mineral IVs. He gave me similar IVs. Juicing, cleansing, nutritional supplements, a nearly perfect diet, prayer, and physical therapy helped my bones and other injuries heal.

After following this regimen for about nine months, what my hand surgeon said would be impossible became real—a fully restored, fully functional hand. He had told me I'd never use my right hand again and that it wasn't even possible to put in plastic knuckles because of its poor condition. But my knuckles did indeed re-form primarily through prayer, and function of my hand returned. A day came when he told me I was completely healed, and though he admitted he didn't believe in miracles, he said, "You're the closest thing I've seen to one."

The healing of my hand was indeed a miracle! I had a useful hand again, and my career in writing was not over as I thought it would be. My inner wounds were what seemed severest in the end and the hardest to heal. Nevertheless, they mended too. I experienced healing from the painful memories and trauma of the attack and the wounds from the past through prayer, laying on of hands, and deep emotional healing work.

I called them the *kitchen angels*—the ladies who prayed for me around their kitchen table week after week until my soul was healed. I cried endless buckets of tears that had been pent up in my soul. It all needed release. Forgiveness and letting go came in stages and was an integral part of my total healing. I had to be honest about what I really felt and willing to face the pain and toxic emotions confined inside, and then let them go. Finally, one day after a long journey—I felt free. A time came when I could celebrate the Fourth of July without fear.

When I look back to that first day in the hospital after many hours of surgery, it's amazing to me that I made it. My hand was resting in a sling hanging above my head. It was wrapped with so much stuff it looked like George Foreman's boxing glove. My face was black and blue and my eyes were red—no whites—they were completely red. A maintenance man came into my room for a repair and did a double take. He asked if I'd been hit by a truck! I felt like I had. As I lay there alone with tears streaming down my face, I asked God if He could bring something good out of this horrific situation. I needed something to hang onto. My prayer was answered. Eventually I knew my purpose was to love people to life through my writing and nutritional information to help them find their way to health and healing. If I could recover from all that had happened to me, they could too. No matter what anyone faced, there was hope.

I have a juice recipe called "You Are Loved Cocktail" on page 162. I named it that because I want you to know that you are loved, that I send you my love between the lines of this book and with the juice and raw food recipes. There is hope for you, no matter what health challenges you face. There's a purpose for your life, just as there was for mine. You need to be strong and well to complete your purpose. You can be greatly served by a positive mind and an optimistic attitude. To that end *The Juice Lady's Living Foods Revolution* can facilitate abundant health to help you live your life to the fullest and to finish well.

My hope is that this book will truly spawn a revolution in the way you think about food and what you choose to eat and drink. And it's my hope that all Americans will change the way they think about food. That will transform health care in America. It will save billions of dollars and millions of lives. This is the true meaning of preventative medicine. The revolution has begun. My prayer is that it will continue with you.

Chapter 1

The Living Foods Revolution

Eat food you love that loves you back...
and you will find the love of your life!
—Raw Chef Avi Dalene

Living foods. They're foods that are *alive*—raw (not cooked) and filled with life. They're also called raw foods or live foods. You can plant them, pick them, sprout them, or simply eat them. In each case—you get life! That's because life comes from life. These foods are your "true north," your path home to health in a jungle of dietary havoc, contaminated food, and abounding confusion about what and how to eat.

What constitutes human nourishment that blesses us with abundant health? Is it the antibiotic-laden, growth-hormone-laced flesh of stressed-out factory-farm animals? How about pasteurized milk products with their denatured protein and damaged fats? Is it cooked or processed vegetables saturated with pesticides and preservatives? Maybe it's designer foods with "good health promises." Perhaps it's the long line of prescription pills coming out of the thunderous jaws of manufacturing plants.

My dear friends, we've been duped—completely led astray—by marketing campaigns. Good health is the result of consuming whole, unprocessed, clean food with a large percentage of that being raw and alive. These foods are chock-full of nutrients, water, and fiber that flush away toxins, waste, and "sludge" from our cells and intercellular fluids. They help us prevent disease. They alkalize our body and help us restore our pH balance. And they give our cells vital light rays of energy to help them communicate more effectively.

How did we lose our way—from pure, whole food to processed, packaged, chemically sprayed industrialized fare—in such a short period of time, considering that for millions of years we ate whole and mostly living foods?

A stroll down memory lane reveals that ramped-up marketing campaigns, clever slogans, and interesting commercials hooked a nation more than half a century ago on money-making products that changed America's thinking about food—forever.

The vegetable oil industry went into full swing during World War II when tropical oils, which were among the healthiest oils on Earth for cooking because they didn't oxidize easily, couldn't make it across the oceans. Well-crafted advertising campaigns touted the benefits of vegetable oil. Wesson cooking oil was recommended "for your heart's sake." They also ran an ad in a prominent medical journal describing it as "cholesterol depressant." Mazola ads said, "Science finds corn oil important to your health." And Dr. Frederick Stare, head of Harvard University's Nutrition Department, encouraged Americans to consume corn oil—up to one cup a day—in his syndicated column.[1]

When the war ended, tropical oils were vilified so that the vegetable oil companies could retain their market share. Was this refined oil our answer to curing the increase in heart disease that followed the war? Research since then has exposed quite the opposite: consumption of those oils is one of the culprits behind heart disease. We now know that oils made from polyunsaturated fatty acids (PUFAs), such as corn, soy, safflower, and sunflower oil, actually contribute to heart disease because they oxidize easily and can *cause* plaque buildup in the arteries. It is insightful to note that the Wynn Institute for Metabolic Research in London studied people who died from heart disease and found that the fats responsible for clogging the arteries of these people were 26 percent saturated fat and 74 percent PUFAs. Rather than implicate saturated fats, they more accurately pointed to PUFAs—the fats found in polyunsaturated vegetable oils—as the primary suppliers to aortic plaque formation. This research group suggested that people avoid these oils completely.[2]

A New Generation of Food and Beverage Products

Cooking oils weren't the only thing to change during this time. Carbonated beverages were also first marketed to the American public shortly after World War II, and by the early 1960s dozens of companies like Coca-Cola were competing for shelf space for their diet and sugar-filled sodas. Marketers promoted their way into our homes with jingles such as, "Zing! Coca-Cola gives you that refreshing new feeling!" Their message? To be part of the hip new generation of young people, you must drink Coke. Chemical sugars such as calcium cyclamate, saccharin, and aspartame replaced white sugar in diet soda with the promise of weight loss. Diet sodas were promoted to diabetics as sugar-free options to popular sugar-packed sodas.

But wait. Do diet sodas really help us prevent weight gain or diabetes? Their promises fall short. The San Antonio Heart Study—a twenty-five-year community-based study carried out at the University of Texas Health Science Center at San Antonio—found the exact opposite to be true. Their research showed that the more diet sodas a person drinks, the greater their chance of becoming overweight or obese. Added weight is a strong risk factor for the *development* of type 2 diabetes. Sharon Fowler, a faculty associate for the San Antonio Heart Study, put it this way: "On average, for each diet soft drink participants drank per day, they were 65 percent more likely to become overweight during the next seven to eight years, and 41 percent more likely to become obese."[3] On top of creating the opposite effect for weight loss and diabetes, these drinks are full of unhealthy chemicals so potent that they can rust nails.

The 1950s also saw the emergence of another new phenomenon in American eating habits: fast food. In 1955 Ray Kroc opened his first McDonald's franchise in suburban Chicago. His advertising slogan—"The All American Meal." It was a fifteen-cent hamburger (four cents extra for cheese), ten-cent fries, and a twenty-cent milk shake. This cheap, kid-friendly combo was served to families as a speedy, twenty-five-second meal-to-go. But was it the "all American" answer for something quick to eat?

What Morgan Spurlock's 2004 film *Super Size Me* revealed was that these fast meals are anything but a healthy all-American choice or a meal to make you happy. For the month of February 2003 Spurlock ate only McDonald's food for three meals a day. He also got no exercise. In the film he documents the dire effects this diet had on his physical and psychological well-being. Within five days Spurlock gained 10 pounds and experienced depression, headaches, and lethargy. By the time the month-long binge was over, the thirty-two-year-old Spurlock had gained 24 pounds. His doctors warned him that he had done irreversible damage to his heart. It took him almost fifteen months to lose the weight he gained.[4]

Since the release of Spurlock's film, McDonald's has stopped super-sizing meals and has added some healthier fare to their menus. But some of the old favorites remain. A close look at the ingredients in their popular Chicken McNuggets—the only "chicken" some kids ever eat—reveals that not everything has been given a nutritional makeover. Here's a complete list of the ingredients in a Chicken McNugget, as posted on the McDonald's website:

White boneless chicken, water, food starch-modified, salt, seasoning [yeast extract, salt, wheat starch, natural flavoring (botanical source), safflower oil, dextrose, citric acid], sodium phosphate, natural flavor (botanical source). Battered and breaded with: water, enriched flour (bleached wheat flour, niacin, reduced iron, thiamin mononitrate, riboflavin, folic acid), yellow corn flour, bleached wheat flour, food starch-modified, salt, leavening (baking soda, sodium acid pyrophosphate, sodium aluminum phosphate, monocalcium phosphate, calcium lactate), spices, wheat starch, dextrose, corn starch. Prepared in vegetable oil (Canola oil, corn oil, soybean oil, hydrogenated soybean oil with TBHQ and citric acid added to preserve freshness). Dimethylpolysiloxane added as an antifoaming agent.[5]

There's obviously a lot more in a McNugget than breaded fried chicken. As this list of ingredients reveals, it also includes a mix of corn-derived fillers (most corn is genetically modified, which is abbreviated as GMO), natural flavorings (often a code word for MSG), leavening agents, dextrose (sugar), and chemicals such as TBHQ and dimethylpolysiloxane. Dimethylpolysiloxane is an anti-foaming agent, which is a type of silicone that is used in cosmetics and other goods like Silly Putty. And tertiary butylhydroquinone (TBHQ) is a synthetic antioxidant preservative that is a common ingredient in processed foods and chewing gum (one of the highest). It is also found in varnishes, lacquers, pesticides, cosmetics, and perfumes to reduce the evaporation rate and improve stability.[6]

A third change in the way Americans eat also came about during the postwar era: prepackaged breakfast cereals. Tony the Tiger made his debut in the 1950s and became an instant hit as the face and voice of Kellogg's Frosted Flakes. In 1957 a popular breakfast cereal ad read, "Wheaties may help you live longer." And Cap'n Crunch and his crew generated mega-sales for Quaker Oats' popular cereals.

Billions of boxes of dry cereal have been sold since such ads danced, sang, and talked their way into our lives. Children as well as adults—even many who are health conscious—eat boxed cereals thinking that they are healthy choices. But let's consider some facts. These cereals are manufactured by means of a process called *extrusion*. First, a liquid mixture called a slurry is created with the grains. Then it's put in an extruder—a machine that forces the slurry out of a little hole at high pressure and temperature. The shape of the hole turns the mixture into the various cereal shapes we're all familiar with: little o's, flakes, animals, shreds, or puffs.[7]

Paul Stitt delves into the extrusion process in his book *Fighting the Food Giants*, explaining that this process destroys most of the nutrients in the grains, such as the fatty acids and even the synthetic vitamins added at the end. However, according to Stitt, the worst part is that extrusion turns the amino acids into toxic matter. The amino acid lysine is especially denatured during extrusion. Stitt also points out that this is how *all* boxed cereals are manufactured, even the ones sold in health food stores. One of the most alarming aspects of extrusion that Stitt warns about is that whole-grain extruded cereals are probably more dangerous than cereals that are not made from whole grains. Why? Because whole grains are higher in protein, and it is the proteins in these cereals that are the most compromised by this process.[8]

You may remember this line: "Wonder bread helps build strong bodies eight ways." (Later it became twelve ways.) In my opinion, the ad should have read, "Wonder Bread helps tear down bodies eight ways." Wonder Bread and other smooth white breads get their soft texture from refined wheat flour. Refined wheat flour has had the natural fiber removed from it because whole grains go rancid rather quickly due to the high oil content in the bran. Refining makes bread that has an extended shelf life, but it no longer gives us much nutrition. And the breads have gotten fluffier and fluffier through the years with hybrid grains that have more and more gluten, created specifically for this purpose. (This is one reason so many people are gluten intolerant today.) These high-starch grains that are made into fluffy breads along with other refined flour products like pasta and pizza crust are targeted as one of the primary contributors, along with sugar, to obesity, diabetes, and heart disease.

Unfortunately, there's more from the 1950s to add to our list of unhealthy eating habits. It was 1954 when Swanson introduced the first TV dinner in an aluminum tray—turkey, cornbread stuffing, gravy, sweet potatoes, and peas. The American family moved from the dinner table to trays in front of the television and started watching TV families interact rather than talking with their own family members while they ate.

It permanently changed the way Americans ate. American families lost the treasure of eating, laughing, sharing the day's events, and praying with the family. We also lost real, whole food made with human hands.

The TV dinner marketing slogans were all about convenience and ease. American women were encouraged to buy the dinners so they could: "Have dinner ready. Prepare yourself. Touch up your makeup. Put a ribbon in your hair."[9] More than 10 million TV dinners were sold in the first year.[10]

Is the ease and convenience of frozen and packaged meals worth it? Many people now consider such meals very unhealthy—too much sodium, monosodium glutamate (MSG), additives, unhealthy fats, not enough vegetables, and no live food, along with aluminum that contributed to heavy metal toxicity (today it's plastic toxicity). If it hadn't been for Julia Child, we may have ended up in worse shape than we are today. Julia persuaded American women to go back to the kitchen and prepare real food.

THE GREEN REVOLUTION AND DESIGNER FOODS

In 1960 we saw the introduction of "miracle seeds"—improved varieties of wheat, corn, and rice, which dramatically increased the crop yields of American farmers. Through the use of pesticides, irrigation, and genetic engineering, these miracle seeds doubled or tripled harvests on the same size plots as previous harvests. The seeds and growing practices quickly spread to farmers in other countries with the hope that they would help end world hunger.

This dramatic increase in crop production was called the "Green Revolution." It was a revolution without a doubt, but far from *green*—which has come to mean buying organic, purchasing foods locally, and promoting sustainable farming and animal husbandry (compassionate care for domestic animals). The hybrid seeds and genetically engineered crops gave us wheat with more gluten so manufacturers could make fluffier bread as I just mentioned, which caused allergies and gastrointestinal problems like Crohn's disease, colitis, and irritable bowl syndrome. Pesticides killed bugs, but it also killed songbirds; it's wiping out our bee population, and it's contributing to cancer and other diseases in humans. In the end, it has killed many of us. (Studies show there is an increased incidence of cancer among farmers, indicating the impact that pesticides have on the human body.[11]) And we must ask ourselves why birds and fish are mysteriously dying by the thousands. Are they the "canaries in the coal mine"? Are we next?

Then along came "designer foods" concocted by food scientists, promising specific health benefits, belched out by big factories, but most often devoid of life-promoting ingredients. They led us astray with their "good health promises" that didn't deliver what they said. As a whole, people are sicker than ever before in history.

Well, this ends our stroll down memory lane. As you can see, we can't trust the jingles, commercials, and marketing ads. They gave us slogans like "Reach for a Lucky instead of a sweet!" And, "More doctors smoke Camels." Here's the truth: we've been the human guinea pigs for decades. We continue to learn, often too late, that many popular products have made us sick, caused deaths, and took our money to boot!

Do you want these people guiding your food choices?

There's a little voice inside calling you home—away from the clamor and spin of the big companies with clever marketing slogans and foods designed to hook you to crave more unhealthy stuff—to the simple goodness of the earth, free of chemicals, genetic tampering, and the fluff that's killing you. The voice is calling you to compassionate eating, sustainability, and supporting local organic farmers. It's time to rethink your perception of food and to discover that you are not too busy to make the time to prepare whole, living foods. You're too busy not to. It's time for a *revolution* in the way you eat and the way you think about food. If you return to nature's living bounty, you can heal your body and mind along with the earth.

Donna Experienced Positive Results in Four Days!

I experienced immediate results physically and mentally in just four days with Cherie's diet. The first day I replaced my morning cup of coffee with white tea and a glass of The Morning Energizer juice. The flavors are amazing. I noticed my normal raging hunger and nausea from coffee on an empty stomach disappeared. I felt a little hungry later, but it was a much different and a very mild feeling. After the first day, I no longer had to take antacids daily and my stomach stopped bloating. I slept more peacefully than I have in a long time. I'm feeling more energy and am calmer than I can remember. When I went grocery shopping, I viewed rows of processed foods, coffees, creamers, cheeses, cookies, cakes, ice creams, and chips. The normal diet choices looked empty and terrible to me. I am simply thrilled with the new me, and I will never return to the diet that was quietly creating illness in me. Thank you with all my heart.

–Donna

I HAD A DREAM

Dreams have often been my teacher. A few months ago I had an insightful sequence of images while sleeping. In the dream, I was in a room with a number of birds that had the freedom to fly and perch where they wished.

I noticed they were all getting sick. So the first thing I checked was their food and water bowls. There was the culprit. The water was not clean, and their food bowls were full of only hulls—the life-giving nourishment had been removed from the seeds. I then saw a large bird make its way to a food bowl. It was weak and sick, and most of its feathers were gone. As soon as it started eating, a big bird flew in and began pecking on its back, drilling a hole in its flesh. I was horrified and tried to beat off the bird of prey with some papers in my hand. It was to no avail. I woke up—deeply disturbed. I knew this dream was significant; it portrayed the state of affairs for many people in our nation.

Americans eat food with little or no nourishment—burgers, fries, hot dogs, sodas, doughnuts, milk shakes, pizza, pasta, packaged foods, fluffy bread sandwiches, low-fat products, and frozen dinners. This food is less nourishing than the birds' hulls in my dream. Then we get sick. We go to the doctor and complain about our ailments. Rarely does anyone ask us what we are eating and drinking. And would it matter? Many of the doctors and nurses seeing us are eating the same things. We go for early-detection tests for various diseases and call that prevention. (What about learning about the lifestyle that helps us to not get sick in the first place? That is true prevention.) When we complain about an ailment, rather than getting to the root cause, we're given prescription drugs that often cause different symptoms, for which we're given additional prescription drugs.

Eventually we get so weak and sick that we, like the sick bird in my dream, have holes drilled in our flesh through surgeries and procedures. To top if off, some of our prescription drugs are found to cause serious problems and even death. Lawyers file lawsuits against the drug companies that manufactured those drugs and win big settlements; most of the money goes to the attorneys. Those drugs are taken off the market and new ones replace them.

I looked with interest at the dream scene where I was trying to beat off the bird of prey with papers. I believe the papers represent my books. I keep writing to expose lies and herald truth. For those who never read my books, my message is to no avail, and the "birds of prey" in our society continue to victimize the weak and sick people and make them weaker, sicker, and more dependent on prescription drugs.

But you're different. You bought this book and are learning truth. For those who have listened and acted in the past, their lives have been changed. I get e-mails and calls continually telling me wonderful stories of healing and hope regarding weight loss and health improvements—this represents thousands of people.

Weight Loss With Health Rewards

I want to share with you the great news! I have lost 11 pounds since starting the coconut-juicing plan three weeks ago. I am off the coffee and sugar addiction cycle and making new discoveries. I feel so good and healthy. My body and skin agree with the recipes. My mental focus is improving, and the dark circles under my eyes are disappearing! I have a good balance of natural energy and cannot believe the blessings in life that I am experiencing each day. I am beyond happy with my new habits and look forward to many more articles, books, classes, and your next adventures. Thank you so much for sharing.

—Chaley

What the Living Foods Revolution Can Do for You

The Juice Lady's Living Foods Revolution is a book based on a lifestyle program I created that involves juicing every day and eating a large percentage of your food while it is still "living," which means uncooked and unprocessed plant foods. These living foods "love you back" by giving you a plethora of life-giving nutrients. That equates to higher energy levels, weight loss, detoxification, mental clarity, increased vitality, and inner peace. But unlike most raw food programs, the Juice Lady's living foods lifestyle program doesn't toss out all cooked food. You can even include a few organic, pastured animal products if you wish. This lifestyle is about choosing pure, whole foods with an abundance of that fare being *live*—raw, juiced, blended, gently warmed, and dehydrated.

Raw green vegetables are emphasized because they have served as the basis of nearly all life on this planet. They're key to our life. I've known this for a long time, but I couldn't get enough of them into my diet to really make a big difference—until I started juicing about a quart a day that included lots of greens. I rotated a wide variety of greens such as Swiss chard, collards, curly kale, black dino kale, kohlrabi leaves, dandelion greens, romaine lettuce, parsley, and spinach, combined with cucumber, celery, lemon, and a carrot or two.

Juicing this wide variety of produce gives us a powerhouse of vitamins, minerals, enzymes, phytonutrients, and biophotons. These foods help to lower estrogen in a woman's body and decrease the chance of contracting breast cancer—something I've always been concerned about since my mother died of breast cancer when I was six years old. Raw foods, which are rich in antioxidants, also help the body remove toxins, thus helping to keep us from getting ill.

Since the beginning of human life, mankind has eaten mostly raw, living foods in season. It is only in recent decades that we have begun eating highly cooked and processed stuff. When we look at other cultures whose people have continued eating their traditional diets, we do not see any significant incidence of diseases such as cancer, heart disease, stroke, diabetes, and morbid obesity that have become pervasive in Western society.

Transformation of Avi

While riding my bicycle to work on July 2, 2001, I was hit by a car. And even though I was wearing a helmet, I sustained a traumatic brain injury. I went through extensive therapies of various kinds, and while they all worked together to make me into the person I am now, [I believe] it is the organic, raw vegan cuisine and transformational super foods that have created and maintained the most healing I have experienced thus far. I have been raw a bit over four years now. Recently, alone at the beach by a fire pit with a box full of papers and memorabilia, I had the funeral for the old me. I left the beach with an empty container and a clean slate to create the life that is calling me.

—Raw Chef Avi Dalene

In our super-sized society where cooked and processed food is served in abundance, living food is a wise choice because it's hard to overeat raw foods. Fresh vegetable juice is amazing in that it offers us many nutrients that are so satisfying that most people lose their cravings.

There are some great benefits of a living foods lifestyle if you're trying to drop a few pounds. Many people say they don't get hungry for quite a while after they drink freshly made vegetable juices. A living foods diet may help you lose weight more quickly, and it can help stabilize your weight once you arrive at your desired goal so that you don't end up gaining it all back. So, even if you consume the average three thousand plus calories per day, chances are you'll just naturally consume fewer calories when you juice because you won't be as hungry. And you can lose weight more quickly and keep those unwanted pounds off with the living foods lifestyle. But the best part is that many people report that weight loss is just secondary to all the other incredible health benefits they experience.

Living foods provide your body with high-energy fuel, so you don't become fatigued throughout the day. Even if you eat a hearty-sized meal of living foods, you won't feel like you need a nap afterward. Further, many people have found that having a glass of fresh veggie juice midmorning or midafternoon is an excellent pick-me-up to keep them mentally alert and energized for hours.

A diet that is made up of 60 to 80 percent raw foods is a live foods diet, because the majority of the foods are eaten in their natural state. Living foods are high in enzymes, which are important to the body because they help in converting vitamins and minerals to energy. Indeed, enzymes are needed for every chemical reaction that takes place in the body. No mineral, vitamin, or hormone can do its work without enzymes. Plant food enzymes work in the digestive system where they predigest foods and thus spare the pancreas and other digestive organs from having to work so hard to produce excess enzymes. Eating living foods, especially vegetables, sprouts, wild greens, fruits, nuts, and seeds, is the healthiest for the human body. Truly they can transform you from the inside out.

A Wonderful Journey of Restoring Health!

Your book is helping me start a wonderful journey of restoring health and stability. I am becoming more familiar with what is beneficial for my body and important foods that are high in alkalinity.

—Linda (not real name)

What if certain diet modifications could increase your chance of living a healthy, youthful life—free from drugs and surgery—well into your eighties, nineties, and possibly beyond? Would it be worth trying?

By switching to a living foods diet, many people have helped their bodies heal from life-threatening diseases such as cancer, heart disease, and diabetes. And many people have reversed the aging process and become trim and fit. Consuming plenty of raw foods re-creates your body inside out. It transforms even your face. Do you want a natural facelift? Eat lots of living foods (and take vitamin C). These are the keys to rejuvenated skin, supporting collagen, and your passport to vibrant health and high-level wellness! They assist your body right down to the DNA with the raw materials that fuel your cells. Lively cells construct a lively body. Healthy cells create vibrant health. They'll help you live your life to your full potential.

THE ABUNDANT LIFESTYLE

Most Americans live a suboptimal existence—mediocre health, low energy, depression, lack of joy, poor memory, poor sleep, and a variety of aches, pains, and ailments. Good health and joyous living are your birthright. You can move toward this quality of life every day if you choose the right lifestyle.

Starting today, you can transition to the living foods lifestyle so you can live the abundant life. As I mentioned before, aim for 60 to 80 percent of your food raw, but even if you just make half of your diet raw, you've made a great improvement. Most live food programs are all or nothing. I've talked with many people who say, "I can't go 'all raw' with my lifestyle." So they forget the whole thing. But when you know that you can have some leeway, it's encouraging to take steps, even baby steps, toward a healthy living foods lifestyle.

Here's how a "living foods day" might look: Drink two 12- to 16-ounce glasses of raw vegetable juice, or make one glass of juice and have a green smoothie, preferably one in the morning to get you energized and one in the afternoon to keep you going. Eat one or two large salads or servings of raw veggies or a raw energy soup. You could choose a piece of low-sugar raw fruit or some raw veggies for a snack. To that you can add about a quarter of your food cooked. If you have an illness or disease, then it is recommended that a larger percentage of your food should be raw (juiced or blended if you have significant digestive issues) and that you occasionally spend a day or two just drinking fresh vegetable juice (juice fasting) to help detoxify your system.

Have you noticed that when you have a day where you eat mostly cooked foods, with very little live food, you want to eat more and more? I experienced that recently. I was served mostly cooked foods at two different events in one day—all whole foods, but about 90 percent of it cooked. At the end of the day I was still hungry. It was 9:00 p.m., and I wanted something else to eat. My body was craving live foods. A little glass of juice did the trick—the urge inside was gone. This is where fresh vegetable juice is so amazing. It's very satisfying. When you feast on raw juices, you can experience the single most effective short-term antidote to cravings, fatigue, and stress available.

Many people call or e-mail to say they feel so much better since they have started on the Juice Lady's living foods lifestyle. I recently received a call from a woman who said those exact words. She has noticed a tremendous amount of energy since starting the living foods and juice program a week before. Prior to that, there were times when she didn't even want to leave the house for days because she was so fatigued. Now she feels like getting out and doing things all the time.

So what's going on?

Raw juices and living foods are packed with a cornucopia of nutrients, including *biophotons*—those light rays of energy the plants get from the sun. When we cook food, those beautiful rays of energy are destroyed or shrink way down. Professor Fritz-Albert Popp and Dr. H. Niggli are two researchers who have found that the light energy in biophotons is an important aspect of food. The more *light* a food is able to store, the more beneficial the food. Naturally grown fruits and vegetables that are ripened in the sun are strong sources of light energy. Numerous minute particles of light—biophotons, the smallest units of light—make their way into our cells when we eat these foods. They provide our bodies with important information and control complex processes such as ordering and regulating our cells.[12]

When you drink a tall glass of fresh veggie juice and your day is focused on more live foods than cooked or processed fare, your whole internal environment changes. As you consume more living foods, you require fewer calories because biophotons help rev up the mitochondria of your cells—the little energy furnaces that pump out ATP (adenosine triphosphate, the energy that is used by cells). They also feed your DNA, which stores about 90 percent of the biophotons found in your cells. Because biophotons carry biological information of the plant into your body, it's kind of like getting a software download or having a computer technician take over your computer remotely to fix things you can't begin to correct. Just as the computer tech fixes errors on your computer, the biophotons help to fix errors that have taken place within the body.[13]

Voilà! You start feeling better, lighter, and more energized as time goes on. Your sleep improves, and you may need less of it. Your mind becomes more alert and creative. No longer will you find yourself in a disorganized fog because biophotons help your mind and body to come alive. You will experience more mental energy, and your creativity improves as well because of the electrical stimulation of the biophotons. (Could this be the boot for dementia or early Alzheimer's disease?) Your metabolism also ramps up, and you burn more calories helping you get fit with greater ease. And in the process, your overall health improves. Symptoms of poor health, ailments, and chronic diseases begin to heal. Your whole life changes!

Juicing Helped When Nothing Else Worked

My husband is a medical doctor. I was an artist. We are very active in our faith and for years participated in foreign missions. We have been everywhere—from the slums of Mexico to the war-torn Congo. Being physically fit and active was and is necessary for such trips. I would carry about 30 pounds on my back and walk five hours into Ecuador's Amazon rain forest to deliver school supplies to remote villages. I had to be able to handle the weight, heat, and terrain.

While in the Congo, even after taking all the precautions and shots, I was bitten by a bug, and my health was never the same. At first my husband thought I had malaria. Then I lost the use of my hands. Being a sculptor, that was devastating. I saw many doctors and spent thousands of dollars on tests. My symptoms escalated. I was tested for multiple sclerosis, Lyme disease, and many, many other things. During this time I lived either on the sofa or in my bed. Actually, I was not living. I was simply existing. Just the simple act of walking was extremely painful. My internist deducted that I had toxic levels of mercury (from old tooth fillings) and lead (from sculpting clay), chronic fatigue syndrome, fibromyalgia, food allergies, and a liver that wasn't functioning efficiently. I took twenty-five pills per day.

I endured IV chelation, colonics, and all sorts of painful and debilitating treatments without lasting improvement. I started seeking specialists in other states. One specialist said I had *Candida albicans* and multiple allergies. He recommended shots twice a week. Monthly I drove eight hours to see him. After that year, I could see no improvement but was suffering from adverse reactions to the medications. In talking with him about it, he told me I had to endure the reactions to gain the benefits. But I didn't see any benefits, so I stopped the shots.

That drove me from the medical field to homeopathic medicine. I was told that I had parasites, so I did the parasitic cleanses that were recommended. That helped a little, but I still wanted my life back. I started driving twelve hours one way to see a specialist who reported that my body still was not absorbing nutrients. I did the Master Cleanse and all sorts of other cleanses. I started eating organically. I was able to function and my pain subsided somewhat, but I remained hungry all the time.

Recently, a friend heard Cherie speak, and she recommended her juice book [*The Juice Lady's Turbo Diet*]. Since getting her book, I've been juicing about two weeks, and it has already made a tremendous difference in my health. My pain has decreased. My brain is not as foggy. I don't need as much sleep. And my skin has improved.

Juicing has helped me more than anything I've tried. Thank you for helping me to live again!

—Natalie

What Living Foods Offer You

- *Alkalinity.* Most Americans are slightly acidic because most of the American diet (animal products, grains, sugar and sweets of all kinds, coffee, black tea, sodas, sports drinks, and junk food) is acidic or turns acidic when it's digested. This causes a host of problems from weight gain to joint pain. The body tends to store acid in fat cells to protect delicate organs and tissues. It will hold on to fat cells, even make more fat cells, to protect you. But a living foods diet, which is dominated with fresh vegetables, vegetable juices, sprouts, seeds, and nuts, provides an abundance of alkalinity. This neutralizes the acids, and the body can let go of fat cells. Many people report that their body also got rid of pain—all sorts of pain throughout the body—when they began eating a living foods diet.

- *Hydration.* One of the things lost when you cook food is the water content. Our bodies are about 70 percent water. Live foods contain lots of water. Approximately 85 percent of many fruits and vegetables is water, so eating raw fresh produce is a wonderful way to obtain water. Plenty of water in our system equates to enzymes being able carry out their metabolic work, and the easier it is for vitamins and minerals to be assimilated into our cells. The more live energy the water holds in the form of biophotons, the better the individual cells function and the higher the quality of your health.

- *Superior protein.* Though not a complete protein, raw plants offer quality amino acids. Cooking denatures the proteins in our food—they coagulate, making them difficult to assimilate. The heat disorganizes their structure, leading to deficiencies of some of the essential amino acids, whereas eating live foods offers amino acids in their best state.

- *Abundant vitamins.* Many vitamins are destroyed when food is cooked or processed.
- *Biophotons.* Plants release biophotons, which can only be measured by special equipment developed by German researchers.[14] These light rays of energy that plants take in from the sun energize our bodies and help our cells communicate more efficiently. Heat and processing destroy them.
- *Greater strength, energy, and stamina.* Dr. Karl Elmer experimented with a raw food diet for top athletes in Germany. He saw improvement in their performance when they changed to an entirely raw food diet.[15] After eating raw food, rather than feeling fatigued or sleepy, most people feel energized. Also, most people eating a high raw food diet experience a more restful sleep and require less of it.
- *Better mental performance.* Your memory and concentration should be clearer. You should be more alert, more creative, and think more logically.
- *More enzymes—improved digestion.* Enzymes are important because they are the catalysts of nearly every chemical reaction in our bodies. Vitamins and hormones need enzymes to do optimal work. Live foods contain a good mix of enzymes, called food enzymes. But when food is heated above 105 degrees, enzymes are destroyed, which forces our digestive system to work harder than it should. This can result in partially digested fats, proteins, and starches.
- *Reduced risk of disease.* A diet rich in raw vegetables and fruit has been shown to lower your risk of cancer and other diseases. Also, according to a study published in the *British Medical Journal*, eating fresh produce on a daily basis has been shown to reduce your chance of death from heart attacks and related problems by as much as 24 percent.[16]

Increase the Micro-Electric Potential of Your Cells

When we eat live foods, our entire bio-terrain operates in peak performance. *Biological terrain* is the system of a cell plus the surrounding environment. It's comprised of fluids, vitamins, minerals, trace elements, enzymes, waste, and microorganisms. When our internal environment becomes overloaded with toxins, waste, and pathogens like fungi, molds, viruses, or bacteria, when it is deficient in essential nutrients or is too acidic or too alkaline, our cells' vitality is diminished and our immune system is overworked. Then we become susceptible to fatigue, ailments, and diseases.

Raw foods and juices cleanse the body of stored wastes and toxins, which interfere with the proper functioning of the cells and organs. They provide an abundance of vitamins, minerals, enzymes, phytonutrients, biophotons, and antioxidants that increase the micro-electric potential of each cell. This improves the body's use of oxygen so the muscles and brain are energized. A healthy, vibrant bio-terrain is fundamental to optimal health. This allows our cells, organs, and systems the best chance to do the jobs they were designed to do. A living foods lifestyle can help you achieve this vibrant interior. With a healthy biochemistry, our bodies can deal with stress and challenges far more effectively. It is only when we put congesting, nutrient-depleted, toxic food into our bodies that we tear them down and promote disease. A living foods diet leads to healing and vibrant health.

Live to Your Full Potential

Secretariat, also known as Big Red, was one of America's heroes and a racing legend—winner of the Triple Crown. He set new race records in two of the three events in the series—the Kentucky Derby and the Belmont Stakes. They still stand today. He ran for the shear pleasure of running. But he lost the Wood Memorial. No one had noticed the abscess in Big Red's mouth, which may have kept him from running to his full potential and from his stunning future.[17]

What about you? Is there a physical condition that's keeping you from being your best or living your full potential? There was for me. Chronic fatigue syndrome and fibromyalgia had me sidelined—as you know if you read the introduction. Had I not found the juicing program that changed my life, I would not be writing my eighteenth book, presenting numerous classes and workshops, appearing on scores of television and radio shows, and accepting speaking engagements around the country for numerous groups and organizations.

Do you ever feel like you're just going through the motions of life, existing rather than living out your dreams and purpose? That can change. You can be so supercharged with health that you live a life of joy and have clarity of mind, and peace of soul. When you care for your body well with the kind of diet recommended in my *The Juice Lady's Living Foods Revolution*, you will have emotional stability and a stronger immune system. You'll be able to deal with stress better than ever before because your nerves won't be on edge with caffeine and sugar. And your willpower will strengthen—a weak body often equates to a weak will.

It may seem too simplistic—that what you eat could have such a profound impact on your health. Owners of thoroughbred racehorses know the importance of a superior diet—good hay and quality grains including oats, mineral salts, and vitamins. You wouldn't catch a racehorse owner giving a horse even one little "treat" of bad food, if they're smart. We're not that different from racehorses. If we want to win the races of our lives, we need a great diet—one that provides quality and energy, one that will take us to the end of our course.

My friend Steve Cesari, former CEO of the $100 million company Trillium that created the Juiceman juicer, and the company where I became the Juice Lady, just released his book *Clarity*. He's passionate about health and juicing. He juices every day. In *Clarity* he shares the story of a friend that offers a great illustration for us about eating right. His friend was in a hurry to get to a soccer game. He needed gas on the way and had to stop quickly to fill the tank. But on his way home, the car broke down. As it turned out, he was in such a hurry that he didn't even realize he'd put diesel fuel in his new Audi. This caused $6,000 worth of damage, and he had to replace the catalytic converter and a number of other parts.[18]

Unknowingly, many Americans put the "wrong fuel" in their bodies over and over again. It's amazing that they can keep going as long as they do. It would be a blessing if it only cost people who "break down" $6,000 to repair the damages.

Remember, every journey begins with the first step. It takes more than a couple of weeks to see a profound difference, although many people report significant improvements in just a few days. Give the living foods lifestyle six months at least and then evaluate. If you haven't noticed profound changes, then you're the first one I've encountered to say that. You should be feeling so much better that you'll never want to go back to your old lifestyle. And you can be on your way to living your potential to the fullest.

Chapter 2

Juicing for a Healthy Lifestyle

Let juice be your medicine, and your medicine be your juice.
—Author unknown

I'M GOING TO give you details on raw foods in just a few chapters, but first I want to cover one of the simplest ways to boost your vegetable intake and increase your raw foods all at the same time: drink more juice. It's a great way to get the vital nutrients your body needs quickly from whole, fresh organic vegetables and fruit.

Plus, statistics show we're not eating enough of these life-giving plants. One study conducted in 2009 showed that only 26 percent of adults surveyed ate three or more vegetable servings a day, which included counting a tomato slice and a lettuce leaf on a burger as a vegetable serving. That was only half the percentage that public health officials had hoped for.[1]

Dr. Joseph Mercola, author of the nation's top natural health newsletter, says he's "firmly convinced that juicing is one of the key factors to giving you a radiant, energetic life, and truly optimal health."[2]

Have you ever considered that juicing could change your life?

If you read my story in the introduction, you know how it changed mine. In chapter 1 you also read an overview of why living food, which includes raw juice, works so well to give you vibrant health: it supplies an abundance of nutrients that satisfies the body's nutritional needs.

There are many cofactors wrapped up in a glass of fresh veggie juice. Cofactors include vitamins, minerals, enzymes, and other elements. Fresh veggie juice is also a great source of biophotons—those light rays of energy that emanate from raw plants and that are lost when they're cooked or processed.

Researcher of biophotons Dr. Fritz-Albert Popp has suggested that, at least in part, the light inside all biological organisms must originate from the foods that are eaten. When you eat plant foods, the biophotons are thought to assimilate right into your body's cells.[3] These light waves convey valuable information used in critical processes throughout the body. There's an indication that they feed the mitochondria—the little power producers of our cells that produce ATP (adenosine triphosphate), a cell's energy "fuel."

This means that when you drink raw juices, fatigue takes a hike. You actually feel like working out and getting things done. And the antioxidants raw juice delivers helps detoxify the body. Toxins can cause weight gain and make it difficult to lose weight, along with contributing to illness, fatigue, and aging.

Juicing Made a Big Difference in Estelle's Health

I am thirty-one years old and have a beautiful family with a gorgeous husband and three children under the age of five years, including a newborn. A few months ago my sister visited Los Angeles. She has severe psoriasis and was looking for something to help. She found your book *The Juicing Lady's Guide to Juicing for Health* and brought it back for all of us to read and try. It was a huge success. Not once through our winter season here in Australia did any of us get the flu or a cold. At the time I was pregnant. I have always suffered with lung problems, but I can honestly say that I, along with my four-year-old son, who is also prone to lung infections and illness, were both healthy the whole time. We have had heaps of energy, and our skin looks clear and refreshed. We have bought your book for other members of our family who are suffering from cancer. It's been a true blessing.

I want to personally thank you for researching, writing, and being a living example of a conqueror. What you have done and been through has helped so many of us and given us the tools to create a healthy life and be the best we can be. I love the God aspect of your story and that you acknowledge how God has been your source; with His help you have made so many people happy and blessed.

—Estelle

Now that you know in theory just how effective juicing is for vibrant health, I want you to experience it firsthand. I'd like to help you get started on your living foods lifestyle with some guidelines for juicing and choosing a good juicer. I'll also give you answers to some frequently asked questions along with plenty of tips to make this a very easy part of your life.

Study Reveals We Need Eight Servings of Fruits and Veggies a Day

A recent study conducted with over 300,000 participants was published January 19, 2011, in the *European Heart Journal.* It revealed that people should consume eight servings of fruits and vegetables per day to significantly reduce risks of fatal heart disease.

Researchers at the University of Oxford analyzed data from a heart study involving 313,074 participants (average age of fifty-four) from ten countries. They collected information about their food habits and other lifestyle factors, including smoking and exercise. The average intake was five portions of fruits and veggies in most countries that participated in the study.

The researchers found that participants who consumed eight or more servings of fruits and vegetables daily reduced their risk of dying from ischemic heart disease (IHD) by 22 percent over those who ate three portions. The results also showed that each additional portion of fruits and vegetables consumed reduced risks of fatal IHD by 4 percent.[4]

Earlier studies have indicated that if everyone ate even five daily servings of fruits and vegetables, 15,000 lives could be saved annually. Think about what would happen if we ate eight or more servings. Juicing can go a long way to help us get at least eight servings.[5]

Super-Hero Vegetable Juices!

Dark leafy greens

Greens offer the nectar of life! Include them often in your juice recipes. They'll love you back every time! There are so many leafy greens to choose—collards, Swiss chard, curly kale, black dino kale, spinach, lettuces such as romaine and green leaf, watercress, parsley, beet greens, dandelion greens, and kohlrabi leaves. These vegetables are among the healthiest choices you can make for juicing.

Because of their high magnesium content and low glycemic index, green leafy vegetables are also valuable for persons with type 2 diabetes. One study revealed that an increase of just one and one-half servings a day of green leafy vegetables was associated with a 14 percent lower risk of diabetes.[6] Further, the high level of vitamin K in greens helps to promote the production of osteocalcin, a hormone that anchors calcium inside the bone and increases both insulin secretion and sensitivity; it also boosts the number of insulin-producing cells while reducing stores of fat. One study found that the risk of hip fracture in middle-aged women was reduced significantly by consuming vitamin K-rich vegetables. The *American Journal of Clinical Nutrition* reported, "Women who consumed lettuce one or more times per day had a significant 45% lower risk of hip fracture than women who consumed lettuce one or fewer times per week."[7]

Green leafy vegetables are also rich in beta-carotene, which can be converted to vitamin A in the body as it is needed. Greens contain nutrients that help immune function. And green vegetables are a very good source of iron and calcium. However, Swiss chard, beet greens, and spinach are not considered good sources of calcium due to their high content of oxalic acid, a natural compound that interferes with the absorption of calcium. This does not mean that you should avoid eating them, because they are rich in many nutrients such as chlorophyll, magnesium, and vitamin K, but rather include them with other greens that are rich in absorbable calcium such as collards, kale, turnip greens, parsley, and watercress.

Dark-green leafy vegetables are rich in lutein, zeaxanthin, and other carotenoids needed in the lens of the eye and macular region of the retina. They help protect the eyes against both cataracts and macular degeneration, two major causes of blindness in older people. Lutein and zeaxanthin also reduce the risk of certain types of cancer, such as breast and lung cancer. And they may also contribute to the prevention of heart disease and stroke.

A Swedish study reported that eating three or more servings a week of carotene-rich vegetables cut in half the risk of stomach cancer, the fourth-leading cause of cancer in the world.[8] A higher consumption of green leafy vegetables has also been shown to significantly decrease the risk of breast and skin cancer.

Quercetin, a bioflavonoid also found in leafy green vegetables, has antioxidant and anti-inflammatory activity and has exceptional cancer preventative properties. Quercetin also blocks substances involved in allergic reactions.

Garlic

Does garlic breath keep you from eating garlic? Here's an answer: juice it up! And include some parsley, which helps you avoid "garlic breath." You'll be getting a multitude of cancer-fighting properties with garlic's active ingredient allicin. Cooking destroys this phytochemical, so eat or juice it raw. It may also help improve your iron metabolism because the diallyl sulfides in garlic help increase production of a protein called ferroportin, which moves iron into circulation. It is also a source of selenium, which is important for the immune system.

Garlic can help to lower blood pressure. Red blood cells use the sulfur-containing molecules in garlic, known as polysulfides, to produce a substance known as hydrogen sulfide (H_2S). This substance helps blood vessels expand and keeps blood pressure from rising.

Garlic also facilitates weight loss. Obesity is a chronic state of low-grade inflammation; therefore, the anti-inflammatory benefits of garlic may be very beneficial for weight loss. Research suggests that garlic may help to regulate the number of fat cells that are produced in the body by inhibiting the conversion of our fibroblastic cells, called preadipocytes, into full-grown fat cells, known as adipocytes.[9]

Garlic is also famous for its antibacterial and antiviral properties. It's a natural antibiotic with broad-spectrum antimicrobial activity that works against many types of bacteria and fungi. Garlic enhances the immune system by promoting phagocytosis—a process whereby immune cells engulf and digest bacteria, viruses, fungi, and other foreign material. And it helps to stimulate other immune cells, such as macrophages and T-cells, to fight bacterial and viral infections. It is very important to strengthen immune cells because they also gobble up cancer cells.

Wheatgrass juice

The liver must filter impurities from the bloodstream—all the car exhaust, paints, cleaners, solvents, preservatives, pesticide residues, drugs, alcohol, and other toxins we encounter almost daily must pass through the liver. This gunk can significantly tax this hard-working organ. Add a diet high in fat, which the liver must emulsify with bile, and a person can experience a host of physical symptoms due to the burden placed on the liver. But along comes wheatgrass juice. Being rich in chlorophyll, it purifies the blood and flushes away toxins such as drug deposits and pesticides. It helps remove heavy metals such as mercury, cadmium, and lead from the body. It also supports red blood cell count. And it helps to lower blood pressure. Further, it is an appetite suppressant and improves metabolism, making it great for weight loss.

And here's a great juice tip: hold wheatgrass juice in your mouth for five minutes; it will help to firm up and tighten your gums. Maybe we should dab this juice on our faces as we drink it!

Dandelion greens

Recently I purchased dandelion greens at our local co-op. They look quite a bit different from the dandelion leaves my grandmother gathered from our backyard to make into tea or add to salad. The store-bought plants live a much more "sheltered life." Wild is heartier and healthier but not available year round. So, thankfully, dandelion greens are turning up more often these days in natural food stores and farmers markets. But if you have them growing in your own backyard, pick them; they're the richest in nutrients because their roots must go deep into the ground to drink up nourishment.

If you gather dandelion greens early, after spring's first warm turn, the leaves and roots are at their height for nutrients. They can be used as a spring tonic and to stimulate digestion and cleanse the liver. They help to restore vitality after a long winter of heavy foods and living indoors. They've been shown to lower blood pressure and support kidney function. They're also a good diuretic. And they help to detoxify the liver and gallbladder. Further, they have antiviral properties, and they help to stabilize blood sugar. (You can read more about dandelion greens and juice in chapter 5.)

Dandelion greens can be juiced alone; however, they taste quite strong. But if you add them to juice recipes, you'll hardly know they are there.

Wild greens

Wild greens like dandelion, nettles, plantain, lamb's quarters, and sorrel, which are often called "weeds" by many people, give us an incredible feeling of satiety. They offer superior nutrition as well as plenty of biophotons. They're also effective in turning off the "hunger switch" by giving you a satisfied feeling. They reduce the desire for starchy foods, which makes them an excellent weight-loss helper. You won't need an appetite suppressant to lose weight when you include a lot of wild green plants in your diet. You can eat a wild plant salad, drink a Wild Green Energy Cocktail (see page 169), or make a wild green smoothie or soup. Like snow in the Colorado sun, the weight will simply start to melt away.

Choose wild greens of your choice to make about 2 ounces of juice and add water or cucumber juice plus a few drops of stevia, some lemon juice, or coconut water. This will energize your body because wild plants contain more vitamins, minerals, antioxidants, phytonutrients, biophotons, and enzymes than cultivated veggies. Consider also that people ate wild plants for several hundred thousand years. Now we eat hybridized and genetically engineered fruits and vegetables, but our physiology is basically still the same. (See chapter 6 for the detrimental aspects of eating GMOs.) Our bodies are crying out for this ancient fuel that we call weeds and that we spray with powerful chemicals that knock them dead before anyone can pick them.

Susan Is Conquering Non-Hodgkin's Lymphoma

Nearly ten years ago my life was turned upside down when I was diagnosed with a form of non-Hodgkin's lymphoma (indolent B-cell). I was told there was not a cure and that chemo was largely ineffective for the indolent form. It was sort of a "watch and wait deal." Immediately after the diagnosis I did two things. I pulled out the dusty old juicer (and used it!) and began to research cancer and natural health. I was determined to find some answers. How did I get here, and how could I regain my health? Years earlier I had introduced juicing and raw foods to the family and especially for our son's health from years of infections and allergies. We slowly returned to the average American diet when his health improved, and we rarely used the juicer.

As a wife and mother of four, I knew I needed to get serious now if I was going to make it. Cancer is radical and demands a radical response! I began a routine of daily juicing and eating mostly raw, whole foods. My energy and prognosis seemed to be improving for a while. Then the cancer started to grow again and into a third area. At this time the oncologist recommended four types of chemo and steroids followed by Rituxan every six months with a 10–15 percent success rate. I still felt I was to build my immune system, not destroy it.

We soon discovered our home was full of deadly black mold. I also learned that my mouth was full of mercury silver fillings and crowns with metal that needed to be removed. I opted for gentler nontoxic materials. Addressing these two areas were key for me, as well as juicing, eating a mostly raw diet, and eliminating sugar.

One of the lifelines for my heath has been the many weeks I've spent at Optimum Health Institute (OHI) in Austin, Texas, for intense times of detoxing, juicing, and the many classes on total person health—body, mind, and spirit. I have seen some tumors go away and others decrease in size through the years as I have applied these health habits.

At the time I started my journey to recovery, the tumor above my left breast was quite sizable and sticking out. I also had tumors on my hip and back. Today, the tumors are 70 percent gone. The breast tumor has shrunk way down. The tumor on my hip is completely gone. The tumor on my back was 4 inches wide and 10 inches long. It had increased in size due to stress from the loss of a loved one. So I went back to OHI and spent about sixteen weeks there. During that time the tumor shrank to 2½ by 4 inches.

I'm alive and thriving instead of dead or dying because of my live foods program. And it's the juicing and raw foods, along with reducing stress and completely avoiding sugar, that are making a huge difference in my recovery.

—Susan

Fresh Juice—a Nutritious Salad in a Glass

Every time you pour a glass of juice, picture a cocktail with a cornucopia of nutrients cascading into your body, promoting health, revving up your metabolism, balancing weight, and increasing vitality. This mélange of nutrients can change your life—completely change your life—as it completely changed mine!

In addition to water and easily absorbed amino acids and carbohydrates, juice also provides essential fatty acids, vitamins, minerals, enzymes, phytonutrients, and biophotons. And researchers are continuing to explore how nutrients found in fresh juice heal the body and help us shed unwanted pounds.

People often ask me if juice isn't just a lot of sugar. That's because they hear this in the media and from doctors. Not the juices I recommend. Fruit juice does contain a lot of sugar—but not vegetable juice. Carrots and beets are higher in sugar, but I recommend you dilute them with cucumber and greens. I also hear people say often that juice has no fiber, so they're avoiding it. Juice has fiber—soluble fiber, which is good for your colon. You do lose the insoluble fiber and *some* of the soluble fiber, so eat a high-fiber diet and complement that with your vitamin-mineral rich juice cocktails. This is a great way to decrease your appetite while increasing your nutrients.

The next time you make a glass of fresh juice, this is what you'll be drinking.

Amino acids

Did you ever consider juice to be a source of protein? Most people would say no. Surprisingly, it does offer more amino acids than you might think. We use amino acids to form muscles, ligaments, tendons, hair, nails, and skin. Protein is needed to create enzymes, which direct chemical reactions and hormones and guide bodily functions. Fruits and vegetables contain lower quantities of protein than animal foods such as muscle meats and dairy products. Therefore they are thought of as poor protein sources. But juices are concentrated forms of vegetables and so provide easily absorbed amino acids, the building blocks that make up protein. For example, 16 ounces of carrot juice (2–3 pounds of carrots) provides about 5 grams of protein (the equivalent of about a chicken wing or 2 ounces of tofu). I don't recommend drinking that much carrot juice because of the sugar content, but that's an example.

Vegetable protein is not complete protein, so it does not provide all the amino acids your body needs. In addition to lots of dark leafy greens, you'll want to eat other protein sources, such as sprouts, legumes (beans, lentils, and split peas), nuts, seeds, and whole grains. If you're not vegan, you can add organic eggs from cage-free chickens and free-range, grass-fed muscle meats such as chicken, turkey, lamb, and beef along with wild-caught fish.

Carbohydrates

Most vegetable juice contains good carbohydrates. The exceptions would be carrots and beets, which have higher sugar content. They should be used in small quantities and diluted with low-sugar vegetable juices such as cucumber and dark leafy greens. Carbs provide fuel for the body, which it uses for energy, heat production, and chemical reactions. The chemical bonds of carbohydrates lock in the energy a plant takes up from the sun and soil, and this energy is released when the body burns plant food as fuel.

There are two categories of carbs: simple (sugars) and complex (starch, glycogen, and fiber). Choose more complex carbohydrates in your diet than simple carbs. There are more simple sugars in fruit juice than vegetable juice, which is why I recommend you juice primarily vegetables, use low-sugar fruit for flavor and a little sweetness, and in most cases drink no more than 4 ounces of fruit juice a day.

Both insoluble fiber and soluble fiber are found in whole fruits and vegetables—both types are needed for good health. It's amazing how many people still say juice doesn't have any fiber. As I mentioned earlier in the chapter, it contains the soluble form—pectin and gums, which are excellent for the digestive tract. Soluble fiber also helps to lower cholesterol, stabilize blood sugar, and improve good bowel bacteria and elimination.

Essential fatty acids

There is very little fat in fruit and vegetable juices, but the fats juice does contain are essential to your health. The essential fatty acids (EFAs)—linoleic and alpha-linolenic acids in particular—found in fresh juice function as components of nerve cells, cellular membranes, and hormone-like substances called prostaglandins. They are also required for energy production.

Vitamins

Fresh juice is replete with vitamins, but heat and processing destroys them. We need these organic substances because they take part, along with minerals and enzymes, in chemical reactions throughout the body. For example, vitamin C participates in the production of collagen, one of the main types of protein found in the body. It's responsible for youthful, supple-looking skin, keeping it from sagging. Fresh juices are excellent sources of water-soluble vitamins like C, many of the B vitamins, and some fat-soluble vitamins such as E and K, along with key phytonutrients such as the carotenes, known as pro-vitamin A (they are converted to vitamin A as needed by the body). They also are coupled with cofactors that increase the effectiveness of each nutrient; for example, vitamin C and bioflavonoids work together synergistically to make each more effective.

Minerals

There are about two dozen minerals that your body needs to function well, and they're abundant in fresh juice. Minerals make up part of bones, teeth, and blood, and they help maintain normal cellular function. The major minerals include calcium, chloride, magnesium, phosphorus, potassium, sodium, and sulfur. Trace minerals, which include boron, chromium, cobalt, copper, manganese, nickel, selenium, vanadium, and zinc, are those needed in very small amounts.

Minerals occur in inorganic forms in the soil, and plants incorporate them into their tissues. As a part of this process, the minerals are combined with organic molecules into easily absorbable forms, which makes plants an excellent dietary source of minerals. Juicing is believed to provide even better mineral absorption than whole vegetables because the process of juicing releases minerals into a highly absorbable, easily digestible form.

Enzymes

These living molecules are prevalent in raw foods, but heat, such as cooking and pasteurization, destroys them. Enzymes facilitate the biochemical reactions necessary for life. They are complex structures composed predominantly of protein and usually require additional cofactors to function, including vitamins; minerals such as calcium, magnesium, and iron; and other elements. Fresh juice is chock-full of enzymes. Without them we would not have life.

All juices that are bottled, even if kept in refrigerators at stores, are required by law to be pasteurized. Heat temperatures for pasteurization are far above the limit of what would preserve the enzymes, vitamins, and biophotons. That's why I don't recommend bottled juices.

When you eat and drink enzyme-rich foods, these little molecules help break down food in the digestive tract, thereby sparing the pancreas, liver, and stomach—the body's enzyme producers—from overwork. This sparing action is known as the "law of adaptive secretion of digestive enzymes," which asserts that the body will adapt or change the amount of digestive enzymes it produces according to what is needed. According to this law, when a portion of the food you eat is digested by enzymes present in the food, the body won't need to secrete as much of its own enzymes. This allows the body's energy to be shifted from digestion to other functions such as repair and rejuvenation.

Fresh juices require very little energy expenditure to digest. That is one reason why people who start consistently drinking fresh veggie juice often report that their digestion and elimination improves and that they feel better and more energized right away.

Phytochemicals

Plants contain substances known as phytochemicals that protect them from disease, injury, and pollution. *Phyto* means plant, and *chemical* in this context means nutrient. There are tens of thousands of phytochemicals in the foods we eat. For example, the average tomato may contain up to ten thousand different types of these nutrients, with one of the most famous being lycopene. Phytochemicals give plants their color, odor, and flavor. Unlike vitamins and enzymes, they are heat stable and can withstand cooking. Some of them, such as lycopene, appear to be more effective when cooked.

Researchers have found that people who eat the most fruits and vegetables, which are the best sources of phytochemicals, have the lowest incidence of cancer and other diseases.[10] Drinking vegetable juices gives you these vital substances in a concentrated form that is easy to assimilate.

Biophotons

There's one more substance abundant in raw foods that is more difficult to measure than the others. It's known as biophotons, which is light energy that is found in the living cells of raw plant foods. These photons have been shown to emit coherent light energy when uniquely photographed (Kirlian photography). This light energy is believed to have many benefits when consumed, such as aiding cellular communication and feeding the mitochondria and the DNA. They are believed to contribute to our energy, vitality, and a feeling of vibrancy and well-being.

Frequently Asked Questions

Now that you know why juice is so good for your health, you may have some questions about juicing. Following are some of the most commonly asked questions:

Why not just eat the fruits and vegetables instead of juicing them?
Always eat your vegetables and fruit. But juice them too! There are at least three reasons why juicing should be included in your lifestyle.

1. You can juice far more produce than you would probably eat in a day. It takes a long time to chew raw veggies. Chewing is a very good thing. It's important for your jaw muscles and your teeth. However, there's only so much time in a day that most of us have for chewing up raw foods. We are no longer hunters and gatherers. One day I timed how long it would take for me to eat five medium-size carrots. (That's what I often juice for my husband and me, along with cucumber; lemon; ginger root; beet; greens such as kale, chard, or collards; and celery.) It took me about fifty minutes to eat them. Not only do I not have that kind of time every day, but also my jaw was so tired afterward that I could hardly move it.

2. You can juice parts of the plant you would not usually eat, such as beet stems and leaves, celery leaves, the white pithy part of the lemon with the seeds, asparagus stems, kohlrabi leaves, broccoli stems, and kale ribs. Not only is that good nutrition, but it is also good economy.

3. Juice is broken down so well that it's very easy to digest. It also spares digestion, meaning that the organs that produce enzymes don't have to work as hard. It is estimated that juice is at work in the system in about twenty to thirty minutes. And, regarding ailments, juice is therapy for this very reason. When the body has to work hard to break down veggies, for example, it can spend a lot of energy on the digestive process. Juicing does the work for you. So when you drink a glass of fresh vegetable juice, all those life-giving nutrients go to work right away to heal and repair your body, giving it energy for its work of rejuvenation.

Don't we need the fiber that's lost in juicing?
It's true that we need to eat whole vegetables, fruit, sprouts, legumes, and whole grains for fiber. We drink juice for the extra nutrients; it's better than any vitamin pill. And regarding weight loss, we drink vegetable juices for appetite control. I also recommend juice as therapy in my book for over fifty ailments: *The Juice Lady's Guide to Juicing for Health.*

Whole fruits and vegetables have insoluble and soluble fiber. Both types of fiber are very important for colon health. The insoluble fiber is lost when you juice; however, soluble fiber is present in juice in the form of gums and pectins. Pectins are especially high in lemons and limes. Soluble fiber is excellent for the digestive tract. It also helps to lower blood cholesterol, stabilize blood sugar, and improve good bowel bacteria.

Don't worry about the insoluble fiber that is lost when you juice. Think about what you are gaining—all the extra nutrition in the juice and plants and parts of plants you'd probably never eat. Then eat a high-fiber diet, and you'll have a great diet. If you're concerned about throwing out the fiber left over from juicing, use it in recipes such as some of the dehydrated cracker recipes you'll find in chapter 8.

Are a lot of nutrients lost with the fiber?

In the past, some people thought that a significant amount of nutrients remained with the fiber after juicing, but that theory has been disproved. The US Department of Agriculture (USDA) analyzed twelve fruits and found that 90 percent of the antioxidant nutrients they measured was in the juice rather than the fiber. That is why fresh juice makes such a great supplement in the diet.

Is fresh juice better than commercially processed juice?

Fresh juice is "live food" packed with vitamins and enzymes. These nutrients are destroyed with heat. That's why I consider bottled juice dead food. Fresh juice also contains that living ingredient, known as biophotons (light energy), which revitalizes the body and even nourishes the DNA; it is also destroyed by heat.

In contrast, commercially processed canned, bottled, frozen, or packaged juices have been pasteurized, which means the juice has been heated and many of the "living nutrients"—vitamins, enzymes, and light energy—are virtually gone. Look at a Kirlian photograph (special type of photography that can capture light rays) of a cooked vegetable or a pasteurized glass of juice, and you'll see very little or no "light" emanating from them. The bottled juice will have longer shelf life, but it won't give your body life.

Pasteurization is required for all bottled juices today, even the juices that are in store refrigerators. This is achieved by heating the juice to a certain temperature (usually between 145 and 250 degrees) to destroy any harmful bacteria, keeping it at that temperature for a certain amount of time, and then rapidly cooling it to a safe storage temperature. This destroys the enzymes, vitamins, and biophotons. You're left with primarily sugar and water. When people say they think juice is high in sugar, they're right if they are talking about bottled fruit juice.

The FDA has ruled that we can no longer buy raw juice in a bottle or package because it could be a source of pathogens. But it might surprise you to know that they have found fungus that is resistant to pressure and heat in processed juices. *Bioscience Research* reported that five commonly sold processed fruit juices (orange, mango, pineapple, tomato, and apple) were found to contain heat-resistant molds.[11] So there's evidence of danger with contamination even from pasteurized juices. (Cranberry is the bottled juice with the least amount of fungi.)

You'll also be getting a wide variety of vegetables and fruit if you make your own juice and choose veggies like kale, beets with leaves and stems, kohlrabi with leaves, collard greens, Swiss chard, arugula, rapini, and mustard greens. These ingredients would rarely or never go into commercial juice. My recipes include all these veggies, plus Jerusalem artichokes, jícama, green cabbage, ginger, celery leaves, black dino kale, and parsley. These sweet, crisp tubers and healthy greens are not found in any processed juices I've seen.

What's Really in That OJ?

The entire orange is put into extracting machines to make commercial orange juice. Enzymes are added to remove as much oil as possible out of the skin, which goes into the juice. That's not good. Orange peel contains d-limonene, which is a useful solvent. Orange oil is used in cleaning products and to kill termites and ants. When it is eaten, it has been found to cause severe reactions in some people. People do eat orange zest, but in very small amounts. Even then it can cause reactions for some people, such as headaches or stomach aches.

But you're not just getting orange oil—that's bad enough, but it's actually the least of your worries. Oranges are a very heavily sprayed crop. The sprays used on oranges contain organophosphate pesticides, which are cholinesterase inhibitors. (Cholinesterase is an enzyme that breaks down the neurotransmitter acetylcholine. Acetylcholine is used specifically to transmit sensory messages.) These pesticides are major neurotoxins—substances that destroy or impair nerve tissue. When they squeeze the oranges in vats, all those pesticides go right into the juice.[12]

Desiring to extract every possible dollar from the orange, they use the leftover orange peel for cattle feed. The dried citrus peel is processed into cakes that still contain plenty of the pesticide organophosphate. The late Mark Purdey in England discovered that these neurotoxins are correlated with symptoms of "mad cow disease" (bovine spongiform encephalopathy [BSE]). When BSE was identified in 1986, Purdey observed that areas where the disease was emerging broadly corresponded with those areas where organophosphate pesticides had been used against the warble fly by being directly applied to the animals' hide.[13] Perhaps not all "mad cow disease" is due to prions (protein particles that have been implicated as the cause of mad cow disease). Or possibly the pesticide that is applied directly to the cattle's hide makes them susceptible to that particular virus. The use of organophosphates is one of the causes of the degeneration of the brain and nervous system in the cow. If these pesticides are affecting the nervous system of the cow this adversely, what are they doing to us?

"Commonly used organophosphate and organochlorine pesticides inhibit acetylcholinesterase at synapses in the somatic, autonomic, and central nervous systems and therefore may have lasting effects on the nervous system," said the authors of a Duke University Medical Center study.[14] Based on these findings, it is highly advisable that you avoid all bottled, frozen, or canned orange juice and only drink freshly squeezed orange juice where the peel is removed.

How long can you store fresh juice?

The sooner you drink fresh juice after you make it, the more nutrients you'll get. However, you can store juice and not lose too many nutrients by keeping it cold, such as in an insulated container, and not exposed to air (covered) or light.

On a personal note: when I had chronic fatigue syndrome, I would juice in the afternoons, when I had the most energy, and store extra juice, covered, in the refrigerator and drink it until the next day when I juiced my next batch. I got well doing that.

How much produce does it take to make a glass of juice?

People often wonder if it takes a bushel basket of produce to make a glass of juice and if they'll go broke in the process. Actually, if you're using a good juicer, it takes a surprisingly small amount of produce. For example, all of the following items, each weighing roughly a pound, yield about one 8-ounce glass of juice: one to two medium to large apples, one large cucumber, or five to seven medium to large carrots. The following each yield about 4 ounces of juice: three large (thirteen-inch) stalks of celery or one large tomato. The key is to get a good juicer that yields a dry pulp. I've used juicers that ejected very wet pulp. When I ran the pulp through the juicer again, I got a lot of juice and the pulp was still wet. If the rpm is too high, or if the juicer has a dull or poor quality blade or is not efficient in other ways, you'll waste a lot of produce, and it will cost a lot of money in the long term. It is far more cost effective to purchase a good quality juicer right from the start.

Will juicing cost a lot of money?

You can figure the cost of a glass of juice is less than a latte. With three or four carrots, half a lemon, a chunk of ginger root, a stalk of celery, half a cucumber, and a fistful of leafy greens, you will probably spend about two to three dollars, depending on the season, the area of the country, and the store.

A new study just released by the USDA Economic Research Service shows just how affordable fruits and vegetables really are. Researchers determined that getting the recommended amount costs only $2 to $2.50 per day. Researchers also found no significant difference between the average prices of fresh and processed fruits and vegetables.[15]

But wait—there are also hidden savings. You may not need as many vitamin supplements. What's that worth? And, you'll probably need far less over-the-counter medications like painkillers, sleeping aids, antacids, and cold, cough, and flu medicines. And then there's time not lost from work. What happens when you run out of sick days? Or if you're self-employed, you've missed out on income each day you're sick. With the immune-building, disease-fighting properties of fresh juice, you should stay well. That's a whopping savings!

How to Choose the Right Juicer

Choosing a juicer that is right for you can make the difference between juicing daily and never juicing again, so it's important to get one that works well for your lifestyle.

People often ask me if they can use their blender as a juicer. You can't use a blender to make juice. A juicer separates the liquid from the pulp (insoluble fiber). A blender combines or liquefies everything that is placed in it; it doesn't separate the insoluble fiber from the juice. If you think it might be a good idea to have all that insoluble fiber like carrot, beet, or celery pulp in your juice for added fiber, I can tell you from experience that it tastes like juicy sawdust. For the clear juice, which is juice you'll enjoy and drink every day, you need a good juicer. Look for the following features:

- *Adequate horsepower (hp).* Look for a juicer with 0.3 to 1.0 hp. Weak-motored machines with low horsepower ratings must run at extremely high rpm (revolutions per minute). A machine's rpm does not accurately reflect its ability to perform effectively because rpm is calculated when the juicer is running idle, not while it is juicing. When you feed produce into a low-power machine, the rpm will be reduced dramatically, and sometimes the juicer will come to a full stop. I have "killed" some machines on the first carrot I juiced.

- *Efficient at extracting juice.* I've used a number of juicers that wasted a lot of produce; there was considerable juice left in the pulp. You should not be able to squeeze juice out of the leftover pulp. Some machines are not efficient, even some expensive ones I've tried, and the pulp comes out wet. I've had people tell me they were spending a lot of money on produce. It often turned out that they had an inefficient juicer.

- *Sustain blade speed during juicing.* Look for a machine that has electronic circuitry that sustains blade speed during juicing.

- *Able to juice all types of produce.* Make sure the machine can juice tough, hard vegetables, such as carrots and beets, as well as delicate greens, such as parsley, lettuce, and herbs. Make sure it doesn't need a special citrus attachment. For wheatgrass juice, you'll need a wheatgrass juicer or a juicer that presses the juice, such as a single or double auger or twin-gear machine, also known as a masticating juicer. Be aware that the machines that juice wheatgrass along with other vegetables and fruit take more time to use. They usually have a smaller mouth, so you have to cut produce up into smaller pieces. Some are more time consuming to clean as well.

- *Large feed tube.* Look for a large feed tube if you don't have a lot of time to devote to juicing. Cutting your produce into small pieces before juicing takes extra time.

- *Ejects pulp.* Choose a juicer that ejects pulp into a receptacle. This design is far better than one in which all the pulp stays inside the machine and has to be scooped out frequently. Juicers that keep the pulp in the center basket rather than ejecting it cannot juice continuously. You'll need to stop the machine often to wash it out. Plus, you can line the pulp catcher with a free plastic baggie from the grocery store produce section, and you won't have to wash the receptacle each time. When you're finished juicing, you can either toss the baggie with the pulp or use it in cooking or composting, but you won't need to wash this part of the juicer.

- *Only a few parts to clean.* Look for a juicer with only a few parts to clean that are also dishwasher safe. The more parts a juicer has and the more complicated the parts are to wash, the longer it will take to clean up and the more time it will take to put it back together. That makes it less likely you will use your machine daily. I just rinse my juicer parts and let them air dry.

- *Slow or quiet juicer*—the next generation of juicers. Two of the most attractive features of this type of juicer are: (1) a low speed technology system, which means it's very quiet (you'll hardly know the machine is on), and (2) it produces a very dry pulp. This is a higher-priced juicer, and you can typically expect to pay between $350 and $400. Because it's more efficient at extracting juice, you may over time pay for the cost of the juicer in savings on produce.

How to Get the Most From Juicing

Juicing is a very simple process. Simple as the procedure is, though, it helps to keep a few guidelines in mind to get the best results.

- *Wash all produce before juicing.* Fruit and vegetable washes are available at many grocery and health food stores. They wash away surface dirt and mold and help to eliminate surface pesticides, but they don't get rid of systemic pesticides in the water and fiber of the plant. Cut away all moldy, bruised, or damaged areas of the produce. Cut off both ends of carrots, ends of large leafy greens such as collards and chard, and ends of celery—actually any end parts or pieces that look brown or dried out.

- *Always peel oranges, tangerines, tangelos, and grapefruit* before juicing because the skins of these citrus fruit contain volatile oils that can cause digestive problems like a stomachache. Lemon and lime peels can be juiced, if organic, but they do add a distinct flavor that is not one of my favorites for most recipes. I usually peel them. Leave as much of the white pithy part on the citrus fruit as possible, since it contains the most vitamin C and bioflavonoids, which together create the best uptake for your immune cells. Always peel mangoes and papayas, since their skins contain an irritant that is harmful when eaten in quantity.

    Also, peel all produce that is not labeled organic, even though the largest concentration of nutrients is in and next to the skin. For example, nonorganic cucumbers are often waxed, trapping pesticides. You don't want the wax or the pesticides in your juice. The peels and skins of sprayed fruits and vegetables contain the largest concentration of pesticides.

- *Remove pits, stones, and hard seeds* from such fruits as peaches, plums, apricots, cherries, and mangoes. Softer seeds from cucumbers, oranges, lemons, limes, watermelons, cantaloupes, grapes, and apples can be juiced without a problem. Because of their chemical composition, large quantities of apple seeds should not be juiced for young children under the age of two, but they should not cause problems for older children and adults.

- *You can juice the stems and leaves* of most produce such as beet stems and leaves, strawberry caps, celery leaves, broccoli stems, kohlrabi stems and leaves, and small grape stems—they offer nutrients too. Discard larger grape stems, as they can dull the juicer blade. Also remove carrot and rhubarb greens because they contain toxic substances. Cut off the ends of carrots since this is the part that molds first.

- *Cut fruits and vegetables into sections or chunks* that will fit your juicer's feed tube. You'll learn from experience what can be added whole or what size works best for your machine. If you have a large feed tube, you won't have to cut up very much.

- *Some fruits and vegetables don't juice well.* Most produce contains a lot of water, which is ideal for juicing. The vegetables and fruits that contain less water, such as bananas, mangoes, papayas, and avocados, will not juice well. They can be used in smoothies and cold soups by first juicing other produce, then pouring the juice into a blender and adding the avocado, for example, to make a raw soup.

- *Drink your juice as soon as you can after it's made.* If you can't drink the juice right away, store it in an insulated container such as a stainless steel water bottle, thermos, or another airtight, opaque container in the refrigerator for up to twenty-four hours. Light, heat, and air will destroy nutrients quickly. Be aware that the longer juice sits before you drink it, the more nutrients are lost. If juice turns brown, it has oxidized and lost a large amount of its nutritional value. After twenty-four hours it may become spoiled. I must add, however, that when I was very sick with chronic fatigue syndrome, I only had enough energy to juice midday. I would store some of the juice for up to twenty-four hours. I got well doing that, so I know the juice had plenty of nutrients even in the stored amount. Melon and cabbage juices do not store well; drink them soon after they've been juiced.

Choose Organic Produce

The recognition of organic foods has increased dramatically in recent years and continues to grow in popularity. Sales of organic foods reach into the billions of dollars each year and continue to increase annually. It appears that an ever-growing number of people want to avoid the billion pounds or more of pesticides and herbicides sprayed onto or added to our crops yearly. That's for good reason! It's estimated that only about 2 percent of this amount actually fights insects and weeds, while the rest is absorbed into the plants and diffused into our air, soil, and water. Please read all the information I've provided in chapter 6 regarding organic produce.

If you are not able to afford to purchase everything organic, avoid the worst offenders. According to the Environmental Working Group, commercially farmed fruits and vegetables vary in their levels of pesticide residue. Some vegetables, like broccoli, asparagus, and onions, as well as foods with thicker peels, such as avocados, bananas, and oranges, have relatively low levels of pesticides (apart from the skin/peel) compared to other fruits and vegetables. Be aware that some vegetables and fruit contain large amounts of pesticide. Each year the Environmental Working Group releases their list of the "Dirty Dozen" and the "Clean Fifteen" fruits and vegetables and rates fruits and vegetables from worst to best. You can check it out online at www.ewg.org.

When organic vegetables or fruit that you want are not available, ask your grocer to get them. You can also look for small-operation farmers in your area and check out farmers markets in season. Many small farms can't afford to use as many chemicals in farming as large commercial farms do. Another option is to order organic produce by mail.

Two Foods That Are Organic "Must-Buys"

1. *Potatoes* are a staple of the American diet. One survey found they account for 30 percent of our overall vegetable consumption.[16] Choosing organic potatoes can have a big impact on your health because commercially farmed potatoes are some of the most pesticide-contaminated vegetables. Also, chlorpropham (CIPC), the most widely used sprout inhibitor, is applied directly to potatoes to prevent sprouting. One animal study found that CIPC had a cytolytic effect (dissolution or destruction of a cell) and reduced intracellular ATP and potassium levels along with causing an alteration in metabolism. (ATP is the energy fuel that powers our cells.)[17] One study found 81 percent of the potatoes tested still contained pesticides after being washed and peeled.[18] The potato has one of the highest pesticide counts of forty-three fruits and vegetables tested, according to the Environmental Working Group. Doesn't this make you think twice before ordering french fries?[19]

2. *Apples* are the second most commonly eaten fresh fruit, after bananas, and they are the second most popular fruit juice, after oranges. But apples are also one of the most pesticide-contaminated fruits. There are between forty and fifty pesticides commonly used on apples. The good news is that organic apples are easy to find and readily available in most grocery stores.

Avoid the "Dirty Dozen"

If you can't afford to purchase all organic produce, you could still avoid the worst pesticide-sprayed offenders by buying only organically grown produce for the top-contaminated list. (Do keep in mind, though, that this choice will not help the plight of farmworkers who fall ill and die of cancer and other diseases at a much higher percentage than the average person.) The nonprofit research organization Environmental Working Group reports periodically on health risks posed by pesticides in produce. The group says you can cut your pesticide exposure by almost 90 percent simply by avoiding the top twelve conventionally grown fruits and vegetables that have been found to be the most contaminated. It has been found that eating the twelve most contaminated fruits and vegetables will expose a person to about fourteen pesticides per day, on average. Eating the twelve least contaminated will expose a person to less than two pesticides per day. The list changes each year. To get the current ratings, go to www.ewg.org.

The Dirty Dozen List (as of 2010)[20]

1. *Celery* has no protective skin, which makes it almost impossible to wash off the chemicals (sixty-four of them!) that are used on crops.

2. *Peaches.* Multiple pesticides (as many as sixty-two of them) are regularly applied to the delicate skins of this fruit in conventional orchards.

3. *Strawberries.* If you buy strawberries, especially out of season, they're most likely imported from countries that have less stringent regulations for pesticide use; fifty-nine pesticides have been detected in residue on strawberries.

4. *Apples.* Like peaches, apples are typically grown with poisons to kill a variety of pests, from fungi to insects. Tests have found forty-two different pesticides as residue on apples. Scrubbing and peeling doesn't eliminate chemical residues that are systemic.

5. *Blueberries* are new on the Dirty Dozen list in 2010. They are treated with as many as fifty-two pesticides, making them one of the dirtiest berries on the market. A friend recently stopped by the road to pick some blueberries. A woman nearby told him that they would come by and spray all the berries in a few weeks before they were picked. She said that when they sprayed the year before, all her goldfish died, but that it didn't hurt her. Sadly, her belief is far from truth; these chemicals hurt everyone.

6. *Nectarines.* With thirty-three different types of pesticides found on nectarines, they rank up there with apples

and peaches among the dirtiest tree fruit.

7. *Bell peppers* have thin skins that don't offer much of a barrier to pesticides. They're often heavily sprayed with insecticides. Tests have found forty-nine different pesticides on sweet bell peppers.

8. *Spinach.* This leafy green can be contaminated with as many as forty-eight different pesticides, making it one of the most polluted green leafy vegetables.

9. *Cherries.* Even local conventionally grown cherries are not safe. In fact, in one survey in recent years, cherries grown in the United States were found to have three times more pesticide residue then imported cherries.[21] Government testing has found forty-two different pesticides on cherries.

10. *Kale.* Traditionally, kale is known as a hardy vegetable that rarely suffers from pests and disease, but it was found to have high amounts of pesticide residue when tested in 2010.

11. *Potatoes.* America's popular spuds may contain as many as thirty-seven different pesticides.

12. *Grapes,* especially imported grapes, run a much greater risk of contamination than those grown domestically. Only imported grapes made the 2010 Dirty Dozen list. Vineyards may be sprayed with various pesticides during different growing periods of the grape, and no amount of washing or peeling will eliminate contamination because of the grape's thin skin. Remember, wine is made from grapes, which testing shows can harbor as many as thirty-four different pesticides. (Only purchase organic wine.)

The Clean Fifteen Food List (as of 2010)[22]

"The Clean Fifteen" harbored little to no traces of pesticides and is safe to consume in nonorganic form. The list includes:

- Onions
- Avocados
- Sweet corn
- Pineapples
- Mango
- Sweet peas
- Asparagus
- Kiwi fruit
- Cabbage

- Eggplant
- Cantaloupe
- Watermelon
- Grapefruit
- Sweet potatoes
- Honeydew melon

What About Mexican Organics?

In the winter, when fresh produce is not available in the United States, we see grocers' shelves stocked with produce displaying Mexican "certified organic" stickers. How many times have you wondered if this is reliable organic produce? In 2007 we imported 3.2 metric tons of vegetables and 1.8 metric tons of fruit from Mexico.[23] But it appears that this produce is as reliable as US grown organics. For a food to be sold in the United States, Mexico, or anywhere else, and to be labeled organic, it must meet all the requirements of the USDA National Organics Program. This means it must be produced without the use of synthetic pesticides, artificial fertilizers, sewage sludge, genetically modified organisms, or irradiation. And it must be certified by a USDA accredited agency to be labeled organic. Certification includes inspection of farms and processing facilities, detailed record keeping of whatever is applied to the land, and, if there's cause for concern, there is water testing. Currently there are fifteen organic certification agencies in Mexico. Plus, the USDA has begun more border inspections to insure food safety.

Supporting Mexican organic farmers is a part of compassionate eating. By purchasing fresh organic produce from Mexico that is not available locally in off seasons, we are supporting small farmers who earn a wage, such as those who sell products recognized as "fair trade," and empower them to stay on their land and remain in their communities rather than leaving home to seek employment.

Chapter 3

Weight Loss on a Mission

In two decades I've lost a total of 789 pounds. I
should be hanging from a charm bracelet.

—Erma Bombeck

WITH THE WORLD Health Organization estimating that by 2015, there will be more than 1.5 billion overweight consumers, incurring health costs beyond $117 billion per year in the US alone,[1] it's apparent that we need to do something differently. We need a new way of life—a revolution in how we eat, one that we adopt for the rest of our lives—not another diet.

Have you repeatedly lost and gained back so much weight you feel like the late Erma Bombeck—you should be hanging from your charm bracelet?

What if you found a weight-loss program that could help you lose weight more effectively than anything you've ever tried? And what if that program didn't involve expensive meals you had to order, pills you had to buy, or anything other than great whole foods you prepare in your kitchen? What if that program helped you look and feel better than ever? And what if it was such an energizing way of life that you wanted to follow it for the rest of your life? Are you interested?

The Juice Lady's Living Foods Revolution is that program. It's a transformative lifestyle that is helping thousands of people lose weight, keep it off for good, and completely revolutionize their health. Donna, who just bought *The Juice Lady's Turbo Diet*, said, "I'm on day four and cannot imagine ever going back to my old eating style." Leslie called to say, "I love this diet. Within three days the pain in my thumb and joints has disappeared." These ladies represent thousands of people who have discovered that the living foods approach to eating offers huge health benefits and is far more than a weight-loss program.

A recent study evaluated surveys of five hundred people on a living foods diet and showed that a high percentage of live foods helped more than 80 percent of the people surveyed lose weight. But this was only the beginning of their health revolution! These people reported marked improvements in immunity (93 percent reported not getting sick with colds and flu). They also cited a change for the better in digestion, allergies, women's issues, chronic illness, mental and emotional well-being, better sleep, and needing less of it. Further, respondents described improvement in all skin conditions surveyed, namely eczema, skin eruptions, dryness, oiliness, and susceptibility to sunburns. There was an overall change in hair, such as increased strength, thickness, and luster, and decreased thinness, weakness, oiliness, dryness, dullness, and dandruff. And they commented on a general enhancement in nail health, such as increased strength and decreased brittleness, chipping, ridges, and fungus.

The number of respondents experiencing body odor after adopting a live foods diet decreased sharply. They also experienced improved eyesight and sense of smell. There was a marked increase in energy and a significant decrease in addictions and use of medications. Results also showed a substantial decrease in allergies in all categories surveyed—food, animal, grasses, trees, pollen, dust, mites, mold, and chemicals. And the vast majority of respondents (87.5 percent) reported better mental, emotional, and spiritual health. Most people attributed the improvements primarily to changing to a living foods diet.[2]

Would you like to experience benefits like these while also losing weight?

So what's really going on when people consume raw vegetable juice and a large amount of live foods? In the pages that follow, I'll tell you about the many unique aspects of the live foods diet and why it works so well for the healthiest weight loss you'll ever experience. This is what I call *weight loss on a mission*—the mission is to help you become healthy, happy, and filled with life, as well as slim and fit. (You'll find more about weight loss in my book *The Juice Lady's Turbo Diet*.)

Weight-Loss Success

[Cherie's book] has provided us with so much information, and we are pleased to have implemented many of the suggested recipes into our diet. Between my husband and myself, we have lost 36 pounds in the past month. Before starting this diet, we purchased a juicer and prepared ourselves for the change in our diet and routine. With the proper planning and knowing that we were going to be very focused on *The Juice Lady's Turbo Diet* as first seen in *[First for] Women* magazine, September 2010, we are so happy with the results. We had concerns, wondering if we could go each day with only juice and raw veggies and hummus until suppertime, but we enjoy this diet, with no hunger issues or concerns. We both feel fantastic and look so much healthier. Our fitness routines have always been part of our lives, but this weight loss and feeling of being so healthy and full of renewed energy gives us such confidence when moving forward and incorporating this diet into our lifestyle. Knowing that we feel so much healthier on the turbo diet is such a huge gift, after years of trying to find the means to be able to lose weight and eat healthy, while at the same time feeling so fantastic.

—Globepro

(posted on *The Juice Lady's Turbo Diet* page on Amazon, November 2, 2010)

Tips for Weight-Loss Success

Cut your calories. Most people lose weight when they embark on a living foods program because they lose cravings for junk food and high-carb foods, which helps you cut a lot of calories. But make sure that you shave off at least 100 calories from your daily caloric intake. All long-term weight studies ever done where people kept the weight off for more than two years showed this simple strategy. And it's very easy to do. Further, 100 calories is such a small amount your body won't be able to tell that you're on a diet. This way your metabolism doesn't slow down, and you naturally lose weight. But don't worry if you're shaving off more than 100 calories a day on a living foods diet, which will probably happen. Your metabolism should not slow down because this style of eating is replete with living nutrients such as vitamins, enzymes, and biophotons that rev up your metabolism.

Eat breakfast. If you think skipping breakfast will cut a bunch of calories from your diet and speed your weight loss, you're mistaken. People who skip breakfast usually eat more for lunch because they're so hungry, and they usually snack more throughout the day. Start your day with a power breakfast—first a glass of raw veggie juice and/or a green smoothie, a nut smoothie, or another living foods dish. Many people say they just aren't hungry after drinking an energizing glass of veggie juice or green smoothie. That may be all you want, but if you're still hungry, follow with some protein such as raw nuts or seeds, raw veggie dip and fresh vegetables, a vegetable omelet, or bowl of old-fashioned steel cut oatmeal. In a study of people who dropped at least 30 pounds,

78 percent said they ate breakfast.[3] Make sure you eat something within an hour of rising, which will boost your metabolism by 10 percent.

Eat healthy snacks. Each day, if you work outside the home, pack healthy snacks in small containers or plastic bags to take with you and keep in your purse, briefcase, or an insulated tote. If you always have healthy diet-friendly snacks like fresh veggies, low-sugar fruit, raw nuts, or seeds on hand, you'll be less tempted to raid the vending machine or grab a few pieces of candy from a coworker's dish. And you won't go home ravenously hungry and eat half a bag of chips or cookies before dinner.

Drink purified water. The next time you feel hungry, drink a glass of purified water and you may not need to eat. Since the hormones in our intestinal tract tell us we're hungry and are very similar to the hormones that let us know we're thirsty, it's often hard to distinguish hunger from thirst. Therefore, we reach for food when we should be reaching for water. Your hunger pangs could be your body's cry for H_2O. Water is essential for burning calories. People who drink eight or more glasses of water a day burn more calories than those who drink less.[4] If you don't like the taste of plain water, add fresh lemon juice. I like lemon and ginger juice added to the water. (My husband and I each drink about a quart of that combination a day.) You may also want to invest in a good water purifier. It's amazing how that improves the taste and purity of the water, which equates to better health.

Go low glycemic. Low-glycemic diet plans, also known as low-carb, are popular for a reason—they get results. High-glycemic foods raise blood sugar levels, cause the body to secrete excess insulin, and lead to the storage of fat. Originally developed as a tool to help diabetics manage blood sugar, the low-glycemic diet has become popular in the weight-loss market largely because it works so well. The *Journal of the American Medical Association* reported that patients who lost weight with a low-glycemic diet kept the weight off longer than patients who lost the same amount of weight with a standard low-fat diet.[5] Low-fat dieting is not good for your body. We need adequate amounts essential fats like omega-3s. Make quality fats about 30 percent of your diet, which will also contribute to satiety—a feeling of satisfaction and that you've had enough to eat.

Debbie Lost Twenty Pounds

I'm another satisfied customer. After a couple of years of Red Bull, tea, and sugar, I went on your Turbo Diet in August. I've lost 20 pounds and lots of inches, mostly in the midsection—4 inches there alone! Thanks so much for the info! This is the best diet ever! I used to be hungry all the time, but now I know I was just never getting the nutrients I needed. Your juice in the morning can sometimes last until the evening meal. Thanks again!!

–Debbie

POWER FOODS THAT GIVE YOUR WEIGHT LOSS A BIG BOOST

In addition to some of the basic steps you can take to achieve weight-loss success, there are specific foods you can add to your weight-loss program that will make a huge difference in assisting your body in burning fat. These super foods can help you succeed and give you super-size health dividends at the same time. Be sure to add them to your living foods lifestyle program.

Green juice: the number one fat cure. In honor of his hundredth show, Dr. Oz served on the set his favorite green juice drink to one hundred people who had lost 13,000 pounds combined. This blend of cucumbers, apple, and leafy greens started a new wave of interest in green juices for weight loss. So why do green juices work so well? Dr. Oz cites the fact that they compensate for the fact that most of us are simply not getting sufficient nourishment from standard diets. He says, "We know we have to have at least five fistfuls of leafy green vegetables and fruit every day, so we make a morning green drink."[6]

There's evidence to suggest that even if we took the time to chew up five cups of green veggies each day, we wouldn't get as much benefit from them as we would from juicing them. The mechanical process of juicing the vegetables breaks apart plant cell walls and makes absorption better than even when the best "chewers" chew their food at least thirty times before swallowing. It has an effect like throwing marbles at a chain-link fence rather than tennis balls; their contents are going to go through the digestive system in a way that "tennis balls" can't.

The juices contain easily absorbed micronutrients that will do more than slim you down—they'll optimize your overall health and wellness. There's science behind the green juices transformative powers and a number of reasons why the juices, along with a high intake of living foods, energize your body, fire up your metabolism, speed slimming, and overhaul your health. Here's the evidence as to why it works.

Magnesium-rich greens ramp up your energy. A British study comparing the metabolism of female twins found that magnesium intake was *the most important* dietary variable that determined adiponectin levels.[7] Adiponectin is a fat cell hormone that promotes insulin sensitivity. This hormone has recently gained attention from researchers because of its regulation of glucose and fat metabolism. Elevated levels of adiponectin are associated with increased insulin sensitivity, and fat burning. Adiponectin also seems to work closely with leptin—a hormone that helps control the appetite and boosts metabolism. As you lose weight on the living foods lifestyle program, this hormone, which is made in fat cells, gets a boost because fresh fruit and vegetables have a positive influence on it. Adiponectin also helps regulate inflammation, which, consequently, helps to prevent gaining weight, becoming a type 2 diabetic, or developing heart disease.

This new study shows very clearly that adequate magnesium is imperative to maintaining adiponectin levels. This means that a deficiency of magnesium, which is common in America, is a clear contributor to the problems people have with weight management. Magnesium also plays a key role in fighting off stress and anxiety, supporting restful sleep, preventing restless leg syndrome, and boosting energy.

Further, magnesium helps prevent fat storage. When magnesium is low, cells fail to recognize insulin. As a result, glucose accumulates in the blood—and then it gets stored as fat instead of being burned for fuel.

Green plants, which are rich in magnesium, are far superior to magnesium supplements because the supplements' particles are a bit large for the body to entirely absorb. (I'm in favor of taking magnesium supplements, if they are needed, but as an adjunct to a magnesium-rich diet.) Green plants take inorganic minerals from the soil through their tiny roots and incorporate them into their cells. They become organic particles that are much smaller and easier for the body to absorb. It is estimated that more than 90 percent of a plant's minerals is delivered to the cells when you juice the greens. So juice up those leaves—chard, collards, beet tops, parsley, spinach—the five highest in magnesium, plus kohlrabi leaves, kale, dandelion greens, dark green lettuce, and mustard greens.

Here's the good news—you'll increase your energy with this high-octane fuel! That means you'll get more done and feel more like working out, so you'll burn more calories and build more muscle.

Can You Get a Tan by Eating Vegetables?

Did you ever think that eating vegetables could give you a healthy tan? It's true. A study led by Dr. Ian Stephen at The University of Nottingham showed that a diet of fruits and vegetables may provide you with a better skin tone than the sun.

The research showed that instead of basking in the sun,

the best way to achieve that golden glow is to munch on fruits and veggies such as carrots, broccoli, spinach, and tomatoes. Dr. Stephen said, "Most people think the best way to improve skin color is to get a suntan, but our research shows that eating lots of fruit and vegetables is actually more effective."

Dr. Stephen and his team found that people who eat more portions of fruit and vegetables per day have more of a golden skin color than those who don't. It's all thanks to phytonutrients known as carotenoids. These substances are antioxidants that help soak up toxins and damaging compounds that get to us from the environment and our food. Toxins are also produced by the stresses of everyday living, and especially when the body is combating illness or disease.

Responsible for the red, orange, yellow, and green coloring in fruit and vegetables, they also give our skin a healthy vibrant color. Dr. Stephen said, "We found that, given the choice between skin color caused by suntan and skin color caused by carotenoids, people preferred the carotenoid skin color, so if you want a healthier, more attractive skin color, you are better off eating a few fistfuls of greens and other fruits and vegetables than lying in the sun."[8]

I would like to point out that you don't need to completely avoid the sun. In fact, unless you have a high risk of skin cancer, it's recommended that you get out in the sunshine without sunscreen for about twenty minutes a day when possible—not to tan, but to help your body produce vitamin D. If you eat plenty of colorful vegetables and fruit, the carotenoids help prevent sunburn, acting as a natural sunscreen from the inside out. If you stay in the sun longer than twenty minutes, it is recommended that you then apply sunscreen, but only use an organic, chemical-free product; chemical-laden sunscreens can contribute to skin cancer.

Enzymes Speed Fat Burning

Our bodies produce enzymes that are used in digesting the food we eat. They can be found in the saliva, small intestine, stomach, liver, and pancreas. These hardworking little catalysts break down proteins, fats, and carbohydrates into fatty acids, amino acids, and forms of glucose that feed your cells.

Enzymes are responsible for a host of reactions in the body. All the minerals, herbs, vitamins, and hormones we take can't do their jobs without enzymes. When your diet is deficient in enzymes from live foods (uncooked, not processed), your body has to work harder to produce the enzymes it needs. If you're deficient, you may experience weight gain, depression, and many other maladies that plague modern society.

Enzymes are truly weight-loss supermen. But these magic bullets start decreasing as we age—by age thirty-five most people see a decline in their enzyme production. Still, we need them for weight loss and good digestion. It's enzymes that assist in the breakdown and burning of fat.

This is where raw foods and juices play a big role.

Living foods come to the rescue—they're packed with enzymes. Eating a high percentage of raw food is important because cooking and processing our food destroys enzymes. To top that off, today's modern lifestyle destroys them in other ways as well. Stress can damage them. Food additives may destroy them. Frequent air travel, coffee, air pollution, food irradiation, and poor sleep all have an impact on enzymes. No wonder we're enzyme deficient as a whole society! This forces enzyme-producing organs, already waning with age, to work overtime on digestion, and it causes your metabolism to take a backseat. That's when you'll see the pounds pack on year by year until one day you know you have to do something fast. When you drink fresh, live juices and eat plenty of living foods, the enzymes they contain kick your metabolism into gear by helping to spare your liver and pancreas from working so hard. Then these organs can focus on their metabolic tasks of burning fat and producing energy. And your digestion will improve. This affects your whole life, your whole being.

The Super-Hero Enzymes

Lipase. Lipase is a fat-splitting enzyme that is abundant in raw foods. It assists your body in digestion, fat distribution, and fat burning. However, few of us eat enough raw foods to get sufficient lipase to burn even a normal amount of fat, not to mention any excess fat. Without lipase, fat accumulates. You can see it on your arms, hips, thighs, buttocks, and stomach. Lipase is richest in raw foods that contain some fat, such as sprouted seeds and nuts, avocado, and fresh coconut meat.

Protease. As your body burns flab, toxins are released into your system. This can cause water retention and bloating. Protease is a digestive enzyme that helps to break down proteins and eliminate toxins. Eliminating toxins is essential when you're burning fat. If your body is storing toxins, it's very difficult to burn fat. But protease comes to the rescue and attacks and eliminates toxins. So, as you can see, it's crucial to have plenty of protease during weight loss. Protease is richest in the leaves of plants. So juice up those green leaves and burn fat. Plus, the greens are also rich in antioxidants that bind up toxins and carry them out of your system so they won't hurt your cells. That means you'll get double action with green juices.

Amylase. Amylase is a digestive enzyme that breaks down complex carbohydrates into simple sugars. It's also present in the saliva. So while we chew our food, it goes to work on carbs. That's why it's recommended that you chew each mouthful of food about thirty times. The pancreas also makes amylase. And amylase is plentiful in seeds that contain starch. (You can juice most seeds of fruits and vegetables.) Its therapeutic use is in regulation of histamine, which is produced in response to recognized invaders to the body. Histamine is a responder in allergic reactions such as hay fever and is what causes hives, itchy watery eyes, sneezing, and runny noses. Amylase breaks down the histamine produced by the body in response to allergens like pollen or dust mites. Some health professionals believe it may help the body identity the allergen as not being harmful so it doesn't produce the histamine in the first place. This is one reason that people on a high raw plant diet often experience improvement in their allergies.

For the most effective approach to increasing enzymes, you may also want to take an enzyme supplement. I especially like an enzyme formula that is taken between meals—it cleans up any undigested particles of food floating around the system and greatly improves digestion. A popular side benefit is that your hair gets thicker and your nails grow stronger. (For more information on these enzymes, see Appendix A.)

Greens Alkalize Your Body and Promote Weight Loss

Many people eat a high-sugar breakfast consisting of foods and drinks like orange juice, toast, jam, honey, sweetened cereal, sweet rolls, doughnuts, muffins, waffles, or pancakes. All this sugar and simple carbohydrates (which turn to sugar easily) promote acidity and cause yeast and fungus to grow. They also produce a lot of acid. Traditional high-protein foods like omelets, cheese, bacon, sausage, and meat promote elevated acid levels in the body as well. Add to that highly acidic drinks such as coffee, black tea, sodas, alcohol, and sports drinks, and you're consuming loads of acid-forming foods throughout the day. Keep in mind that acid-forming food does not mean the state of the food when you eat or drink it but the final ash residue after it is metabolized. As a result of this style of eating, along with not eating enough fresh green veggies and other living foods, many people suffer from a condition known as mild acidosis, which is an out-of-balance pH leaning toward acidity. This means that the body is continually fighting to maintain pH balance.

One of the symptoms of acidosis is weight gain and an inability to lose weight. That's because the body tends to store acid in fat cells and to hang on to those cells to protect your delicate tissues and organs. It will even make more fat cells in which to store acid, if they're needed. To turn this scenario around, it's important to alkalize your body. Greens are one of the best choices you could make because they're very alkaline. And juicing them gives you an easy way to consume a lot more than you could chew up in a day.

To give your body a great start in rebalancing your pH, make 60 to 80 percent of your diet alkalizing foods like green vegetables, raw juices, grasses like barley greens and wheatgrass juice, fresh vegetables and fruit, raw seeds, nuts, and sprouts. Greatly limit or avoid your consumption of acid-forming foods such as meat, dairy products, chocolate, sweets, bread and all other yeast products, alcohol, carbonated drinks, sports drinks, coffee, and black tea.

When pH balance is achieved, the body should automatically drop to its ideal, healthy weight unless you have other health challenges. (But those should also heal over time.) As the acidic environment is neutralized with mineral-rich alkaline foods, there will be no need for your body to create new fat cells for storage of acid. And since the remaining fat is no longer needed to store acid wastes, it simply melts away.

This is also a great way to restore your health. Many diseases such as cancer thrive in an acidic state. Take away the acid, and they don't do as well. An alkaline diet also boosts your energy level, improves skin, reduces allergies, sustains the immune system, and enhances mental clarity.

THERMOGENIC FOODS REV UP YOUR METABOLISM

Thermogenesis means the production of heat, which raises metabolism and burns calories. Thermogenic foods are essentially fat-burning foods and spices that help increase your metabolism. This means that with some of your kitchen staples, you can burn off fat during or right after you eat and increase your fat-burning potential just by eating them. So include these super foods often in your juices and dishes.

Hot peppers. Imagine eating hot peppers and revving up your metabolism enough to lose weight. A study in 2010 found that obesity was caused by a lack of thermogenic response in the body rather than by overeating or lack of exercise. "The animals developed obesity mainly because they didn't produce enough heat after eating, not because the animals ate more or were less active," said Dr. Yong Xu, instructor of internal medicine at UT Southwestern and co-lead author of the study.[9] Another study found that hot peppers turn up the internal heat, which helps in burning calories.[10] You can add hot peppers or a dash of hot sauce to many juice recipes or almost any dish and make it taste delicious.

Garlic. When it comes to weight loss, garlic appears to be a miracle food. A team of doctors at Israel's Tel Hashomer Hospital conducted a test on rats to find out how garlic can prevent diabetes and heart attacks, and they found an interesting side effect—none of the rats given allicin (a compound in garlic) gained weight.[11] Garlic is a known appetite suppressant. The strong odor of garlic stimulates the satiety center in the brain, thereby reducing feelings of hunger. It also increases the brain's sensitivity to leptin, a hormone produced by fat cells that controls appetite. Further, garlic stimulates the nervous system to release hormones like adrenalin, which speed up metabolic rate. This means a greater ability to burn calories. More calories burned means less weight gained—a terrific correlation.

Ginger. This spice contains a substance that stimulates gastric enzymes, which helps boost metabolism. The better your metabolism, the more calories you'll burn. It has been shown to be an anti-inflammatory—inflammation is implicated in obesity. Ginger helps improve gastric motility—the spontaneous peristaltic movements of the stomach that aid in moving food through the digestive system. When the digestive system is functioning at its best, you'll experience less bloating and constipation. It has also been found to lower cholesterol. And ginger is the top vegan source of zinc, which gives a big boost to your immune system. Top that off with the fact that it tastes delicious in juice recipes, and you have a super spice. I add it to almost every juice recipe I make.

Parsley. This dark green herb offers a great way to make your dishes and juices super healthy. Parsley helps you detox because it's chock-full of antioxidants, like vitamin C and flavonoids, and it's loaded with minerals and chlorophyll. It's also a natural diuretic, which helps you get rid of stored water. That means thinner ankles, feet, and fingers. And it improves digestion and strengthens the spleen. You can add a handful of parsley to almost any juice recipe and you won't even know it's there.

Cranberries. Studies show that cranberries are loaded with acids that researchers believe are useful in dissolving fat deposits. When fat deposits settle in the body, they are hard to get rid of, so it's best to get them before they get "hooked on" you. Some studies point out that the enzymes in cranberries can aid metabolism, which gives a boost to weight loss.[12] This tart little fruit is a natural diuretic, helping you get rid of excess water and bloating. Of all the fruits, cranberries rank number two for antioxidant content, which helps detoxify the body. And they promote healthy teeth and gums, fight urinary track infections, improve heart health, and keep cancer at bay.

Kathy, who was featured in my "Holiday Fat Buster" article in the December 27, 2010, issue of *Woman's World*, issue, lost 5 pounds in seventy-two hours drinking a cranberry, pear, cucumber, and ginger cocktail along with following the rest of the turbo juice diet program. Within a week Kathy's tummy was down 5.5 inches—she said she had to keep measuring to make sure it was right. Regarding the turbo juice diet program, she said, "Overall, I had a lot of energy and no hunger."[13]

You can add cranberries to many recipes for a delicious enhancer to your juice drinks and a boost to your weight loss at the same time. If you buy these berries when they're in season, you can freeze a few packages to have on hand for seasons when they aren't available.

Blueberries. A 2010 study found that blueberries can help you get rid of belly fat, thanks to the high level of phytochemicals (antioxidants) they contain. The study also showed that blueberries are helpful in preventing type 2 diabetes, and the benefits were even greater when the blueberries were combined with a low-fat diet.[14] Moreover, blueberries can also help fight hardening of the arteries and improve memory. Make sure you purchase only organic blueberries, since they are on the Dirty Dozen list. (See page 46 for more information.)

Lemons. Adding just a tablespoon of fresh lemon juice to your water, salad, or soup will help ward off cravings, alkalize your body, and keep your insulin levels in check. Hot lemon water with a dash of cayenne pepper is a great way to start your day—it gets the liver, your fat-burning organ, moving in the morning. It's also a natural diuretic and helps clear out toxins from your system. Further, it aids the digestive process and prevents constipation. It can also help alleviate heartburn—just add a tablespoon of fresh lemon juice to water and drink with your meal. Limonene, a compound in lemons, helps short-circuit the production of acid in the stomach—lemons are very alkalizing. Meyer lemons, my favorite, are sweeter and are available in the winter.

One more tip for heartburn: If lemon water doesn't help you, you may not have enough stomach acid. Rather than being too acidic, you may need acid to aid digestion because your stomach is not producing enough. Don't let this confuse you with having slight acidity. Stomach acid is a different factor. You must have strong stomach acid to digest food, but this acid production wanes as we age; after about age thirty-five, it starts slowing down. Try drinking a tablespoon of apple cider vinegar mixed with about 8 ounces of purified water. Apple cider vinegar is quite acidic. If it helps you, that's a sign your heartburn or acid reflux is related to too little stomach acid. In that case, drink apple cider vinegar water with meals and/or take HCL Betaine, which can be purchased at most health food stores.

Conquering Yeast: A Key for Successful Weight Loss

Candida albicans is an opportunistic fungus that is often the link between weight gain, feeling ill, and difficulties losing weight. In fact, yeast overgrowth was linked to an average weight gain of 32.5 pounds in studies at the Fibromyalgia and Fatigue Centers in Dallas, Texas.[15]

Focusing on removing yeast from the body rewards you with a feeling of well-being and steady, sustainable, and healthy weight loss. If the yeast is allowed to continue its growth, it can mutate into a fungus that can spread throughout the body. Unless halted, the fungus will not stop; it can completely destroy your health. In worst-case scenarios, the sufferer may become bedridden because the *C. albicans* fungus can completely drain a healthy body of all energy by pumping it full of toxins (mycotoxins).

Americans have embraced the low-carbohydrate diet for its ability to reduce their waist size when other diets have failed. But an equally important benefit of a low-carbohydrate diet is that it starves yeast of their primary food—sugars. A person with systemic *C. albicans* will often crave sugar and simple carbohydrates because this is the main source of nutrients for yeast. Mood swings, PMS, and depression are associated with the rapid change in blood sugar levels caused by yeast. People complain of gas and bloating that yeast causes by fermenting foods in their intestines. Yeasts naturally release gas just as champagne and beer do. Yeasts also produce alcohol via fermentation, which is absorbed through the gut and may cause symptoms of brain fog, altered behavior, and difficulty concentrating.

Do You Have an Overgrowth of Yeast?

❏ Intense carb cravings
❏ A white-coating on the tongue
❏ Nail fungus, yellowing of nails; athlete's foot
❏ Bloating, diarrhea, constipation, heartburn
❏ Postnasal drip, sinusitis, congestion

- ❏ Regular headaches or migraines
- ❏ Frequent colds or other infections
- ❏ Difficulty concentrating, brain fog
- ❏ Irritability, mood swings
- ❏ Skin eruptions or acne
- ❏ Dry, itchy skin
- ❏ Rashes

Determining whether you have a yeast overgrowth can make a big difference in how you will be able to lose weight and keep it off as well as your overall health. (For an extensive candidiasis written questionnaire, which can help you better determine if you have a yeast overgrowth, see my book *The Coconut Diet.* It also has more than seventy delicious recipes using coconut oil to help you conquer yeast.)

Gabriela Dropped Eleven Pant Sizes

Appearing in *First for Women* magazine's September 2010 issue that featured my book *The Juice Lady's Turbo Diet,* Gabriela's before and after pictures tell the story: she went from 260 pounds to 130. Gabriela shared her story of struggle with weight that had kept her in maternity clothes for twelve years. This mother of four said she knew her habit of starting each day with ten mini powdered doughnuts wasn't helping her, but her cravings seemed uncontrollable. As her belly grew, so did her list of health complaints—yeast and urinary tract infections, joint pain, migraines, dry skin, and lack of energy. "I finally got to the point where I couldn't stand how I looked or felt," she said. "I didn't want to live the rest of my life sick." So after doing research, she cut back on carbs and drank fresh juices made with celery, spinach, and berries. The diet change worked: "I haven't been sick in three years!" she exclaimed. And her size? She shrunk from a size 24 to a size 2.[16]

Chlorophyll Deactivates Systemic Yeast

Molds, fungus, and yeasts (all fungi) are single or multicell organisms that can cause us to gain weight. Yeast cells numbering in the millions can colonize the digestive track. Those who have accumulated higher than normal levels usually will crave carbs—sweets, alcohol, and starches such as bread, potatoes, white rice, crackers, rolls, bagels, pasta, and pizza because the yeasts demand to be fed. And those cravings are often uncontrollable. Eating this stuff leads to bloating and weight gain. A person may also lose muscle strength. If they continue to feed the fungi by eating simple carbohydrates and starches, the whole situation becomes a no-win frustrating cycle—the strength of the fungi increases. More fat is produced. And many health problems worsen.

C. albicans produce a large number of biologically active substances called mycotoxins, which are highly acidic waste products. These toxins are secreted to serve the fungi by protecting it against viruses, bacteria, and parasites. They can get into the bloodstream and produce an array of central nervous system symptoms such as fatigue, confusion, irritability, mental fogginess, memory loss, depression, dizziness, mood swings, headache, nausea, numbness, and hypoglycemia. And these toxins can produce chronic illness, frequently described as "feeling sick all over."

The body has difficulty cleansing fungi spores from the mucous membranes throughout the body and controlling its overgrowth systemically. One of the actions of mucus is to collect and absorb harmful microbes like toxic fungi. An overgrowth can contribute to illnesses like sinusitis and congestion. Under normal conditions these organisms can be controlled, but when the amount coming in or reproducing exceeds the body's systems of control, the accumulations create problems.

Research at Oregon State University has shown that chlorophyll binds to mycotoxins, thus blocking them from entering the bloodstream.[17] This makes the beautiful green juice recipes in chapter 8 potentially life-changing for up to 80 million Americans (70 percent of them women) and men who suffer with an overgrowth of *C. albicans*.[18]

Green juices and savory green smoothies can make a big difference for you if you suffer with symptoms such as chronic fatigue, persistent sinusitis, allergies, carb cravings, and vaginal infections related to yeast overgrowth. The fungi do not like an environment rich in chlorophyll, which is a compound found in plants that is essential to photosynthesis and gives plants their color. Foods rich in chlorophyll make the fungi's job much tougher. It is very alkaline and neutralizes the acidity produced by the mycotoxins. It also binds them, stopping the fungi's destructive cycle. So pour yourself a big glass of green juice and knock the fungi out!

Greens Could Save Your Life

Besides being rich in vitamins, minerals, and chlorophyll, greens could save your life. According to a recent study from Lawrence Livermore National Laboratory (LLNL), consuming a small dose of chlorophyll—found in green leafy vegetables such as spinach, chard, collards, broccoli, parsley, and kale—may reverse the effects of aflatoxin poisoning.

Aflatoxin is a cancer-causing toxic substance produced by mold that occurs naturally in certain foods, including corn and corn products, cottonseed, peanuts and peanut products, tree nuts, and milk.[19]

Probiotics: Weight-Loss Heroes That Help Control Yeast

The composition of microflora, the bacteria in the digestive tract, could help to determine how many calories are absorbed from food. Recent research suggests that these good bacteria can increase metabolism and weight loss. *Nature* reported that overweight people have different microorganisms in the gut than lean people, suggesting that obesity may have a microbial aspect to it. According to the report, when an obese person loses weight, their microbial population reverts back to that of a lean person.[20]

Japanese scientists also discovered that probiotics promoted weight loss. They recruited eighty-seven overweight people who were given 200 grams of fermented milk every day for twelve weeks. The participants were randomly divided into two groups: those whose fermented milk contained *Lactobacillus gasseri* (a probiotic) and those whose fermented milk did not. Significant decreases in body weight, BMI, waist circumference, and hips were observed in the Lactobacillus group but not in the control group.[21]

Probiotics are dietary supplements or foods that contain the kind of good bacteria naturally found in the body. According to Mayo Clinic nutritionist Katherine Zeratsky, "These microorganisms may help with digestion and offer protection from harmful bacteria, just as the existing 'good' bacteria in your body do."[22]

Most people think of yogurt when they consider foods rich in probiotics. But raw vegetables, fresh veggie juice, and fermented foods such as miso and sauerkraut add plenty of good "living" bacteria to the intestinal tract. Keep in mind that cooking kills good bacteria. This is another reason why people on a living foods diet often lose weight.

Two Super Foods That Kill Yeast

There are several foods that will help to lower your yeast levels and get you on track to controlling them. Include plenty of the following foods.

Organic virgin coconut oil. A study in 2007 in the Department of

Medical Microbiology and Parasitology at University College Hospital in Nigeria demonstrated the effectiveness of virgin coconut oil as an antifungal agent that killed *C. albicans.* Researchers concluded that coconut oil destroyed 100 percent of the yeast cells on contact. Specifically, credit goes to lauric, caprylic, and capric acids in coconut oil that worked synergistically to split open the protective outer wall of yeast cells. The dose used was 3 tablespoons daily.[23] Coconut oil can be substituted in place of other dietary fats such as butter or oils.

Numerous animal and human research studies have confirmed that replacing long-chain fatty acids—found in polyunsaturated oils like corn, safflower, sunflower, and soy oil—with medium-chain fatty acids (MCFAs)—found in coconut oil—results in both decreased body weight and reduced fat deposits. This is because MCFAs are easily digested and turned into energy, and they stimulate metabolism. Several studies have also shown that MCFAs can enhance athletic performance.[24]

Another benefit of coconut oil is that it boosts the thyroid gland, helping your body's immune system to function better and aiding in weight loss. (See chapter 4 on thyroid health—a sluggish thyroid is one of the "hidden" reasons behind an inability to lose weight.)[25]

Coconut Oil–Hope for Diabetics

The benefits of coconut oil are good news for the 26 million Americans who have diabetes or prediabetes. This healthy oil provides energy without producing insulin spikes. It also helps stabilize weight gain, which means you're decreasing your chances of developing type 2 diabetes if you add it to your diet.[26]

Raw garlic. Two antifungal actions of raw garlic (cooked doesn't work) have been identified by studies at Putra University in Malaysia:

1. It stops the formation of *hyphae*—long strands that branch off of yeast and enable it to spread.
2. It causes yeast cells to die prematurely.[27]

You need to eat at least one raw clove a day—or juice it with one of the recipes in chapter 8.

Fit and Fab in Record Time

What can ten minutes of brisk exercise do for you? A recent study indicated that ten minutes of vigorous exercise triggers metabolic changes that can last at least an hour. Further, the more fit you are, the more benefits you'll get. Researchers measured biochemical changes in the blood of a variety of people. Metabolic changes that started after ten minutes on a treadmill were still measurable sixty minutes after people cooled down.[28]

At Massachusetts General Hospital, researchers measured biochemical changes that occur during exercise. They found alterations in more than twenty different metabolites. Some of these compounds help you burn calories and fat, while others help stabilize your blood sugar. Some of the metabolites revved up during exercise, such as those involved in processing fat, while others involved with cellular stress decreased.[29]

The best way to burn fat and lose weight is now proving to be short bursts of anaerobic exercise in which you raise your heart rate up to your anaerobic threshold for twenty to thirty seconds and then recover for ninety seconds. This could be fast walking alternating with slow walking. My favorite is an interval class that incorporates both step aerobic and alternate weight-lifting exercises. This short-burst type of exercise can increase your human growth hormone (HGH) level, which helps you sleep better as well as lose weight, improve muscle tone, reduce wrinkles, and increase energy. The longer you can keep your body producing higher levels of HGH, the longer you will experience robust health and strength.[30]

An Exercise Machine for Everyone!

The lymphasizer, also known as the healthy swinger or swing machine, is an ideal alternative or a great addition to an exercise regimen because it will actively move the lymph and blood through the body. You only need to lie down on the floor with your feet in the padded grooves of the machine; it does the rest. It's very beneficial for people with circulation problems in their feet that stem from such things as diabetes or steroid drug use. It's also helped many people who have had lymph nodes removed and experienced problems with swelling. With this machine, you'll have a zero-impact workout that requires no active movement. You just lie on the floor with your feet on the machine's grooves and get the aerobic benefits of a half-hour of exercise in about ten to fifteen minutes.

The lymphasizer provides a simple exercise without applying any stress on the spine, ankles, knees, or other body parts. It will gently rock your body from side to side like the movement of a fish moving through water.

This simple rocking motion maintains a proper energy balance and oxygen supply to the body. Regular use of this relaxing massage movement stimulates your body and achieves relaxation and stress reduction. A sense of well-being arises from the massaging, swing action that is immediately noticeable. Using the lymphasizer before bedtime promotes more restful sleep as well as weight loss.

Though this machine is a great addition for everyone, it can be excellent for the disabled, for anyone with serious knee or ankle problems, those who are very overweight and find other forms of exercise difficult, or for those who for other medical reasons are unable to even bounce slowly on a rebounder.

It is especially important to move the lymph through the system. The lymphatic system has no pump, so exercise is the way we can move this waste through our body so it can be eliminated. I have used our lymphasizer for years. Before one naturopathic doctor (ND) appointment where I had a detox footbath treatment, I spent about twenty-five minutes on the machine. My ND was very surprised at all the lymph in the detox bath at the end of the session. That's when I knew the machine was really working to detoxify my lymphatic system.

A lady contacted me who had had several lymph nodes removed along with a breast lump. She had experienced immense swelling in that breast—to almost double its normal size, making her very uncomfortable. When she started using the lymphasizer, all the swelling went down and her breast returned to normal size. (For more information on the lymphasizer, see Appendix A.)

SLEEP—IT MAY BE A KEY TO YOUR WEIGHT-LOSS SUCCESS

In our frenzy to experience it all, get it all done, manage our universe, and not let a moment escape us, we're missing out on one of our body's most important needs—a good night's sleep. "We're shifting to a twenty-four-hour-a-day, seven-day-a-week society, and as a result we're increasingly not sleeping like we used to," says Najib T. Ayas of the University of British Columbia. We're really only now starting to understand how that is affecting our weight and our health, and it appears to be significant.[31]

A whopping one-third of our population sleeps only six and a half hours or less nightly—far less than the eight hours that many sleep specialists recommend. Will Wilkoff, MD, author of *Is My Child Overtired?*, says the number of overtired patients he sees has soared in the last twenty-five years since he has been in practice because families are trying "to squeeze twenty-six hours of living into a twenty-four-hour day."[32]

Research is showing that there is a correlation between the lack of sleep so many Americans are experiencing and the weight gain that is plaguing our nation. "We've known that people use food as a pick-me-up when they are tired, but now it appears they are hungrier than we realized, and there is a hormonal basis for their eating," says Thomas Wadden, director of the Weight and Eating Disorders Program at the University of Pennsylvania in Philadelphia.[33]

Columbia University studied the sleep habits of 3,682 people and found that those who got by on less than four hours of sleep a night were 73 percent more likely to be obese than those who slept seven to nine hours nightly. Those catching a moderate six hours of sleep a night were 23 percent more likely to be obese. Other studies report that reducing sleep to six and a half hours or less for successive nights causes potentially harmful metabolic, hormonal, and immune changes that can lead to illnesses and diseases such as cancer, diabetes, obesity, and heart disease.[34]

If you've thought sleeping was a waste of time, you don't need to feel guilty about sleeping ever again.

There are hormones that make you hungry and hormones that control your appetite. And research shows they are significantly influenced by how much sleep you get. Here's what studies have revealed:

- Five major appetite-influencing hormones can get out of whack when you don't get enough sleep, which significantly affects how much food you eat.[35]
- When you are sleep deprived, your metabolism can really suffer, which causes weight gain.[36]
- Appetite-suppressing hormones and appetite-stimulating hormones are best regulated when you get seven to nine hours sleep per night.[37]
- You won't tend to crave high-calorie, carbohydrate-rich foods nearly as much when you get adequate, refreshing sleep.[38]
- Sufficient sleep will help you manage your blood sugar more effectively, which helps you manage your appetite. Even one week of sleep deprivation can set off a temporary diabetic effect causing you to crave sugar and other fattening foods.[39]

Sleeping in a few extra minutes has its advantages. Research shows that if you increase your sleep by just thirty minutes per night, your chances of losing weight go up exponentially.[40]

It's apparent that getting plenty of refreshing sleep on a consistent basis, and enough sleep to meet your body's needs, could be far better for your weight-loss goals than diet pills and just as important as working out or eating right.

But what if you want to sleep more and can't? That happened to me a few years ago, ironically, while I was writing *Sleep Away the Pounds*. And just when I was at the point of true despair, I found an amino acid program that turned my sleepless nights into ones of deep, restful sleep again. A urinalysis test pinpointed the excitatory brain neurotransmitters such as epinephrine and norepinephrine that were too high and the calming, sleep-enhancing neurotransmitters such as serotonin and dopamine that were too low. With a tailored amino acid supplement program I was able to bring my biochemistry back into balance enough so that within about three weeks I started sleeping deeply through the night. It was the answer that addressed the root cause of the problem, whereas sleeping pills did not. In fact, sleeping pills made me feel groggy and not at all present during the day, and they did not produce a restful, rejuvenating night's sleep but a weird light sleep where I was easily awakened. (For more information, see Appendix A.)

A Diet of Raw Vegetables Healed Her Lungs

Not too long ago I was diagnosed with pulmonary fibrosis; tests indicated my lungs were white. I was prescribed ten different medications and given five years to live. I was told that by the time I was two to three years into the progression of the disease, I would be in a wheelchair and would not be able to breathe on my own; I would need to be on oxygen. Eventually I was hospitalized with severe edema. All the medicines I'd been given made me feel very ill. So I finally decided that if I was going to die anyway, why take all those medications that added to my physical problems. I quit taking everything. About that time my daughter-in-law persuaded me to go on a diet of mostly raw vegetables that consisted of green beans, carrots, tomatoes, celery, bell peppers, onions, and salads. Within five months I had lost 50 pounds. She finally persuaded me to go to the National Jewish Health Hospital in Denver, which is the leading respiratory hospital in the United States. I had not wanted to go because I thought, "Why go? I'm dying anyway." But feeling better after my vegetable program, I decided I would fly to Denver for further testing. Can you imagine how shocked my husband and I were when the doctor said, "Why are you here? You're not sick; you're going to be fine." There were only a few small spots on my lungs. The only thing I had changed was my diet.

—Ladonna

Chapter 4

Living Foods for Thyroid and Adrenal Health

*In order to change we must be sick and
tired of being sick and tired.*

—Author unknown

COULD POOR THYROID function be making you sick, tired, or overweight? Your thyroid is a key gland that's tied to every other system in your body. When it's out of balance, you're out of balance. The thyroid is a butterfly-shaped gland located at the base of your neck, just below your Adam's apple. Although it weighs less than an ounce, it has an enormous effect on your health. All aspects of your metabolism—from the rate at which your heart beats to how quickly you burn calories—are regulated by thyroid hormones.

A blood test may never indicate that you have a problem with this gland because these tests are designed to identify hypothyroid, not a suboptimal—just-a-bit-below-par—thyroid function. Take the Low Thyroid Health Quiz below, giving yourself a point for every symptom that describes you. If you have a number of the symptoms of low thyroid, chances are that you could benefit by working on your thyroid health with the living foods lifestyle program.

Low Thyroid Health Quiz

Score 1 point for each symptom that applies to you.
- ❏ Appetite problems–severely reduced or excessive
- ❏ Bipolarity (manic depression)
- ❏ Bloating or indigestion after eating
- ❏ Brittle nails
- ❏ Calcium deficiency
- ❏ Carpal tunnel syndrome
- ❏ Chronic mucus in head/nose (thyroid governs mucus production)

- ❏ Coarse, dry hair
- ❏ Cold hands and feet
- ❏ Constipation
- ❏ Decreased sweating
- ❏ Depression
- ❏ Difficulty concentrating
- ❏ Difficulty drawing deep breaths
- ❏ Dry mouth; drinking water doesn't help much
- ❏ Dry, rough skin
- ❏ Elevated cholesterol
- ❏ Emotionally unstable
- ❏ Enlargement of heart
- ❏ Fatigue/lack of energy
- ❏ Feeling of deep gloom for no apparent reason
- ❏ Fluttering in ears
- ❏ Forgetfulness
- ❏ Gasping for air occasionally
- ❏ Grinding teeth during sleep
- ❏ Grooves or ridges in nails
- ❏ Hair loss
- ❏ Heart pain
- ❏ Heart palpitations
- ❏ Hoarse throat
- ❏ Hypertension
- ❏ Impaired heart function
- ❏ Impotency
- ❏ Inability to "drag oneself from bed"
- ❏ Intolerance to closed, stuffy rooms
- ❏ Intolerance to cold or heat
- ❏ Irritability for no apparent reason
- ❏ Left arm weakness
- ❏ Lethargy
- ❏ Light menstrual flow
- ❏ Loss of hair on arms, underarms, legs, eyebrows, scalp
- ❏ Loss of hearing
- ❏ Loss of libido/low sex drive
- ❏ Loss of smell
- ❏ Low body temperature (below 97.6 degrees, resting)
- ❏ Miscarriages
- ❏ Mucus accumulation

❏ Muscle/joint problems—knees, elbows, etc.
❏ Need for fresh air
❏ Nervousness
❏ Numbness in fingers
❏ Occasional stinging in eyes
❏ Pain in diaphragm
❏ PMS
❏ Poor absorption of minerals
❏ Poor digestion of animal products
❏ Poor vision
❏ Premature deliveries
❏ Prolonged or heavy menstrual bleeding
❏ Puffy eyes
❏ Restlessness
❏ Sense of pressure (compression) on chest
❏ Shorter menstrual cycle
❏ Shortness of breath
❏ Shyness
❏ Sleep disturbances
❏ Slow growing nails
❏ Slower heart rate
❏ Sluggish lymph drainage
❏ Spleen or liver problems
❏ Stiff neck
❏ Stillbirths
❏ Swelling—ankles, eyelids, face, feet, hands, lymph nodes, throat
❏ Tendency to cry easily
❏ Tenderness in lower ribs
❏ Thin, peeling nails
❏ Weight gain or difficulty losing weight
❏ White spots on nails (this can also be a zinc deficiency)

A score of 20 points or more may be indicative of low thyroid. Although the thyroid quiz can help you determine your thyroid health, ultimately the best method for diagnosis is clinical evaluation by a physician knowledgeable in thyroid health. I recommend you see a physician who can treat your condition holistically.

Thyroid problems are prevalent in this country, affecting as many as 20 percent of women and 10 percent of men. Many people go undiagnosed. But even for the people who learn that they have an overactive or underactive thyroid, it can be difficult to heal. Nevertheless, it's important to work on healing this gland because a healthy thyroid makes about 80 percent of the T4 hormone and 20 percent of the T3 hormone and traces of T2, T1, and calcitonin.

T4 is the major metabolism hormone and controls many functions of the body. It's converted into T3 in the liver. T1 is thought to assist in the conversion process. If you produce too little T4, or if the T4 you produce is not being properly converted into T3, your whole system goes haywire—you suffer from a variety of symptoms such as low sex drive, fatigue in the morning, and weight gain. If you drastically cut calories to lose weight, calorie deprivation only serves to slow thyroid function further and causes more weight gain.

T3 is critical to your fitness because it sends messages to your DNA to rev up your metabolism and increase fat burning. It helps lower cholesterol, improves memory, keeps you trim, promotes growth or regrowth of hair, relieves muscle aches and constipation, and even helps with infertility in some people.

T2 is known to have a stimulatory effect on the enzyme that converts T4 to T3. It is also effective in promoting liver metabolism and is involved in the activity of the heart muscle tissue. It also affects "brown fat"—the fat that is burned rather than stored in the body. Further, T2 can help in the breakdown of fat, making it an important hormone for weight loss and bodybuilding.

Calcitonin, a protein hormone, slows the release of calcium from the bones; it decreases bone breakdown and increases bone density. It also keeps blood levels of calcium low. There is a higher incidence of osteoporosis among people with hypothyroid, which would make sense since this gland regulates calcium metabolism. A 2007 study shows that calcitonin may protect postmenopausal women from osteoarthritis. In the study, female rats were given salmon calcitonin; they showed less joint damage than those who were given a placebo.[1]

It's important to remember that using prescription thyroid hormone replacement is at times necessary, but it should only be used as a Band-Aid (a temporary solution) while the actual cause of hypothyroid is explored. It's not advantageous to stay on thyroid medication indefinitely even though these hormones may reduce symptoms. It doesn't heal your thyroid gland. In fact, it has the opposite effect—your body will slowly produce less and less thyroid hormones because there are enough hormones in your system. Like your muscles, your thyroid will get weaker and weaker from lack of use. At the same time, you'll produce less calcitonin, and your bones will suffer.

Thyroid Problems: Causes and Contributing Factors

There are many causes of hyperthyroidism (overactive thyroid) and hypothyroidism (underactive thyroid) that are never addressed or treated when diagnosed: things like imbalances in stress hormones or sex hormones, environmental toxins, food allergies, nutritional deficiencies, inflammation, and infections—all of which may be a source of the problem. Also, poor diet can harm the thyroid's ability to make T4 thyroid hormone as well as the cell's ability to convert T4 into the active form T3.

By understanding some of the major contributing factors in hyper- and hypothyroidism, it is possible to correct the problem and heal this gland.

Psychological factors

Not only are we affected by stress, but we're also affected by our responses to the stressors. Actually, our responses are more important because they determine the degree to which our body is impacted by the stress. Personality issues are also important, such as being high-strung, extremely ambitious, aggressive, or angry, which create more stress.

Dietary factors

People who consume too many sea vegetables, iodized salt, stimulants such as caffeine and sodas, or take too much tyrosine may experience hyperthyroidism. On the other hand, excessive consumption of raw cruciferous vegetables (arugula, broccoli, brussels sprouts, cabbage, collard greens, cauliflower, kale, mustard greens, bok choy, radish, horseradish, kohlrabi, turnip, rutabaga, watercress, and rapini) and the mint family (basil, bugleweed, catnip, lavender, lemon balm, marjoram, motherwort, oregano, peppermint, rosemary, spearmint, thyme) can suppress the thyroid gland because they block iodine absorption. This can contribute to hypothyroidism. All these vegetables and herbs are very healthy, however, and should not be eliminated from your diet but rotated with other vegetables. The cruciferous vegetables should be eaten in smaller amounts. The herbs are not of concern because they're usually eaten in small amounts. Cooking can help to deactivate some of the goitrogenic compounds in the vegetables and herbs. Also, soy products (edamame, tofu, tempeh, soy sauce, miso, soy cheese, soymilk, textured vegetable protein) and peanuts are in the same goitrogenic category and block iodine absorption. Additionally, deficiencies of iodine, zinc, and vitamins A, B_2, B_3, B_6, and E can contribute to hypothyroidism.

Toxins

The thyroid is a sentinel organ and is usually one of the first that is impacted by toxicity. According to the Functional Endocrinology Center of Colorado, chemicals such pthalates, flame retardants, bisphenol A, dioxins, perfluorinated chemicals (PFOA), fluoride, perchlorate, thiocyanate, and pesticides can be very disruptive for thyroid function and seriously impact your health. Also, radiation can disrupt thyroid function. Let's take a closer look at several items on this list.

Phthalates increase the flexibility of plastics and are commonly used in shower curtains, medical tubing, and plastic toys. They're also found in personal care items like nail polish and lotion. Phthalates impact thyroid regulation by decreasing thyroid hormone receptor activity. Because of their widespread use and the fact that municipal water treatments don't remove them, they are showing up in drinking water.[2]

Polybrominated diphenyl ether (PBDE) is a flame-retardant chemical used in furniture foam, carpets, upholstery, clothing, toys, draperies, and electronics. This chemical readily accumulates in fat cells and has been linked to a decrease in TSH levels.[3]

Bisphenol A (BPA) is commonly used in polycarbonate water bottles, baby bottles, plastic toys, medical tubing, food packaging, and dental sealants. It has also been linked to disruption in thyroid receptors and thyroid function.[4]

Dioxins, including polychlorinated biphenyls (PCBs), polychlorinated dibenzodioxins (PCDDs), and polychlorinated dibenzofurans (PCDFs), are by-products from industrial processes like chlorine paper bleaching, pesticide manufacturing, and smelting. Have you heard of Agent Orange used during the Vietnam War? Dioxins were part of this toxic biological weapon. Among other things, these chemicals interfere with production, transportation, and metabolism of thyroid hormones.[5]

Perfluorinated chemicals (PFOA [perfluorooctonoic acid] and PFOS [perfluorooctane sulfonate]) used in nonstick cookware, stain-resistant materials, and food packaging have been linked to decreased thyroid hormone levels.[6]

Perchlorate is a by-product of rocket fuel production that has shown up in drinking water, certain fruits and vegetables, and dairy products from cows that eat contaminated grass. It can inhibit iodine absorption, leading to low thyroid function.[7]

Thiocyanate is a chemical found in cigarettes and certain foods, and like perchlorate, it may inhibit iodine uptake and therefore lead to decreased production of the thyroid hormone.[8]

One of the best things you can do to avoid all this is to purchase only organic produce because pesticides sprayed on nonorganic foods often contain estrogenic compounds, which can affect the endocrine (hormonal) system that includes the thyroid. Avoid all plastic water bottles. Purchase a high-quality water purification system. Use an air filter in your home. Cook with only natural product cookware. Choose organic mattresses, bedding, towels, carpets, and fabrics for your home. Clean with eco-friendly, natural products. And choose only fragrance-free, chemical-free, and organic personal care products.

To make sure that you get rid of harmful toxins that have built up in your system, detox your body at least once, but preferably twice, a year. Keep in mind that sweating is the only known way to get rid of plastic toxins, so sauna detox is very beneficial. (See chapter 5.)

Are Nonstick Pans Affecting Your Thyroid?

Ryan Robbins, ND, a naturopathic physician and resident at Bastyr Center for Natural Health, posted an article on Bastyr's website in which he stated, "For several years, synthetic chemicals have been suspected of contributing to thyroid conditions such as hypo- and hyperthyroidism, as well as thyroid cancer. In the United States, 16 percent of women and 3 percent of men will develop some form of thyroid disease during their lives."[9]

Robbins explains that one group of chemicals—perfluorinated compounds (PFCs)—causes great concern. They are used to make nonstick cookware. They're also used in stain-resistant carpeting, rugs, and fabrics; flame-resistant and waterproof clothing; wood sealants; paints; and food packaging.

Two of these PFCs—perfluorooctane sulfonate (PFOS) and perfluorooctanoic acid (PFOA)—cause cancer and lead to hormone disruption and liver damage, according to Robbins. And according to a 2010 report in the journal *Environmental Health Perspectives*, men and women with high PFOA levels were twice as likely to have a thyroid disorder as those with lower levels.[10]

Here is what Robbins recommends (as do I) to avoid exposure to these chemicals:

- Eat only whole food and avoid all packaged, processed foods.
- Avoid slick food packaging like microwave popcorn bags and coated coffee cups.

- Use only stainless steel, glass, or ceramic mugs and stainless water bottles for all drinks, but especially for hot drinks; avoid plastic and Styrofoam cups. Tote your food in reusable glass or ceramic ware.
- Use safer alternatives to Teflon like Thermolon (used in Green Pan cookware), seasoned cast iron, or glass cookware. It's best not to use Teflon at all; when it's heated to 260 degrees, it starts releasing toxic gases into the air we breathe.
- Use only natural cleaning products like baking soda, white vinegar, and vegetable oil-based soaps.
- Avoid all stain-resistant carpeting, rugs, and fabrics, and all fire-retardant and waterproof fabrics, mattresses, and clothing.
- Drink only purified water that has had toxic organic compounds removed.[11]

Living Foods Revolution for the Thyroid

Some foods boost thyroid function, which makes them perfect for hypothyroidism, while others suppress thyroid function, which can help people with hyperthyroidism. And there are certain foods that are best for everyone to avoid for the sake of a healthy thyroid gland and overall health.

The following foods are among the most helpful for restoring thyroid balance whether you have an underactive or overactive thyroid.

- Raw foods—follow the living foods lifestyle program and menu plan
- Fresh raw vegetable juices
- Low-sugar fruit, especially lemons, limes, cranberries and other berries, and green apples
- Raw nuts and seeds
- Seaweed for its rich iodine content (for hypothyroid)
- Chlorophyll-rich green juices such as watercress, collards, chard, kale, kohlrabi leaves, beet greens, and parsley (vary the cruciferous greens with other non-cruciferous greens, such as lettuce, beet greens, watercress, and spinach, if you have hypothyroidism)

Nicole Healed Her Body

When Nicole first came to my group, she had multiple health problems. She was only thirty years old and had hypothyroid, endocrine imbalances, insomnia, and low energy. Inspired to make a difference in her health, she changed her diet to the living foods lifestyle, which included some juicing early on, live foods, and cooked whole foods. Her health completely turned around. I recently interviewed her.

"Before making all the dietary changes, my sleep was horrible," she said. "I had trouble falling asleep. I woke up a lot during the night and had trouble getting back to sleep. I didn't wake up refreshed or energized. I also had thyroid and endocrine system problems. But since your class, I've made some major changes in my diet.

"I used to eat a lot of junk food and drink 2 to 4 liters of soda per day. Now, I haven't touched a diet soda in months. I'm actually enjoying cooking. I like eating vegetables, fruit, whole grains, beans, and some meat. One of my favorite dishes to make is sweet potato and brown rice enchiladas with fresh greens. Some of my other favorite dishes are also very easy to make. For example, I slice an acorn squash in half, bake it, and add broccoli slaw, red pepper strips, ground turkey breast, a dollop of nonfat yogurt, and some fresh herbs and spices. Or how about butternut squash soup: cube butternut squash and roast; purée with coconut milk, curry, cinnamon, and cumin; heat on stove. Then add fresh chopped veggies and throw in some cooked cubed chicken breast and fresh herbs at the end. Homemade pesto is super easy too: blend fresh basil or arugula with fresh garlic cloves, pine nuts, and olive oil. It makes a delicious dip for baby cucumbers, carrot sticks, or mushrooms. Sometimes I take grape tomatoes, garlic cloves, and fresh basil and drizzle with grapeseed oil and a sprinkle of salt and pepper. Roast in the oven for a delicious and healthy appetizer or dinner side.

"Occasionally my husband and I go out to dinner. We usually don't feel so great afterward, so we go right back on our healthy program. The living foods lifestyle has transformed my health. I just got my lab test results from my doctor. My blood work is normal. I still take thyroid medication and bioidentical hormones, but I'm feeling great! I'm now sleeping through the night and wake up feeling refreshed. I have the energy to work out, which I love doing, while I didn't before. My hair is thick and healthy, where it was formerly falling out, thin, and dry. I've experienced great changes in my skin as well. These health changes have given me true passion about nutrition, and I love passing on this information to friends."

—Nicole

Nutrients That Support the Thyroid

The oils

Coconut oil. It was discovered in the 1940s that when farmers used coconut oil to fatten their animals, it made them lean and active instead. Medium-chain fatty acids are known to increase metabolism and promote weight loss. They also appear to help the thyroid gland. People frequently report that when they take 2–3 tablespoons a day of organic virgin coconut oil, their thyroid gland function appears to improve. Other people notice that they don't need as much thyroid medication as they formerly did because their thyroid gland starts functioning better. Some people have reported that they've been able to get off medication completely. Coconut oil is good for medium heat cooking with a smoke point of 350 degrees.

Extra-virgin olive oil. Olive oil is monounsaturated oil that does not oxidize as easily as polyunsaturated oils. It is good for cold foods, dressing, and light sautéing, but it is not good for even medium heat cooking because it has a low smoke point of about 305 degrees.

Iodine-rich foods

It is imperative to provide the thyroid gland with all the nutritional cofactors needed to make thyroid hormone. Iodine is one nutrient that is critical for good thyroid function. Consume more of these iodine-rich foods:

- Sea veggies, kelp, and dulse
- Seafood and fish
- Cranberries (grown in bogs on the coastline, they contain iodine)

Selenium

Selenium may be the "hero" of nutritional supplement thyroid therapies. It is essential for converting T4 thyroid hormone into T3. It may also have the ability to suppress anti-thyroid antibodies in people who suffer from thyroid inflammation or thyroiditis. Reversing a selenium deficiency could, in some people, actually repair thyroid metabolism by increasing the intracellular conversion of T4 to T3. Foods rich in selenium include: seafood, Brazil nuts, barley, red Swiss chard, oats, brown rice, beef, lamb, turnips, garlic, barley, egg yolk, chicken, radishes, and pecans.

Zinc

Zinc is needed for the hypothalamus to stimulate the pituitary gland, which signals the thyroid gland to produce thyroid hormone. Ginger root is one of the best sources of zinc.

Vitamin D

Vitamin D is necessary for thyroid hormone production in the pituitary gland and possibly in binding T3 to its receptor. Vitamin D is a critical nutrient because numerous studies have found that many Americans are deficient in this important vitamin, which also affects bone health and even cancer prevention. If you haven't been tested, it would be wise to get the blood test and know where your vitamin D levels stand.

WHAT TO AVOID

Sugar of all types

Sweeteners can be a big problem for the thyroid gland. Sugar can cause "burnout" for both the thyroid and adrenal glands. Blood sugar changes can also promote diabetes and hypoglycemia, both of which often occur in people with thyroid issues. Some people report increased energy and that their thyroid levels stabilize when they stop eating sweets altogether. Sweets also cause a rise in triglycerides, so avoiding them can help return triglycerides to a normal level.

Goitrogens

Goitrogens are substances that suppress the function of the thyroid gland by interfering with iodine uptake. Following are the goitrogenic foods you should avoid or greatly reduce.

Soy. Soy is one of the most prevalent goitrogens—which means iodine blockers. The National Center for Toxicological Research showed that the isoflavones in soy are damaging to the thyroid in adults and especially worrisome in children because they block thyroid peroxidase.[12] Soy contains estrogenic compounds that can interfere with thyroid hormones and sex hormones, contributing to PMS, cramps, bloating, and menopause symptoms. Some people with hyperactive thyroid find that small amounts of soy (only organic—soy is a big GMO crop) help modulate their thyroid gland. But people with low thyroid should avoid soy altogether—no tofu, textured vegetable protein, soymilk, soy cheese, soy ice cream, tempeh, seitan, miso, or edamame.[13]

One retrospective epidemiological study showed that teenaged children with autoimmune thyroid disease were more likely to have received soy formula as infants (eighteen out of fifty-nine children; 31 percent) compared to healthy siblings (nine out of seventy-six; 12 percent) or control group children (seven out of fifty-four; 13 percent).[14]

Cruciferous vegetables. A family of vegetables known as the cruciferous or mustard family contains goitrogenic chemicals that suppress the thyroid. Some goitrogenic compounds induce antibodies that cross-react with the thyroid gland; others interfere with thyroid peroxidase (TPO), the enzyme responsible for adding iodine while thyroid hormones are produced. Like isoflavones in soy, isothiocyanates in cruciferous veggies appear to reduce thyroid function by blocking TPO. These vegetables include broccoli, cauliflower, spinach, kale, mustard, brussels sprouts, cabbage, bok choy, turnips, rutabagas, radish, horseradish, arugula, rapini, canola, and kohlrabi. Foods and herbs from the cruciferous and mint families are very nutritious, and many have important medicinal properties. Regular consumption of these plants will not lead to underactive thyroid function unless other factors are also involved, particularly iodine deficiency.

Only those who already have hypothyroidism need to be concerned. In these cases, foods from the cruciferous family should be reduced but not eliminated from the diet. Cooking does appear to help deactivate the goitrogenic compounds found in these vegetables. As I stated earlier, spices and herbs from the mint family aren't as much of a concern because they aren't consumed in as large a quantity. However, regular consumption of herbal products containing bugleweed, motherwort, and lemon balm should be avoided.

Other goitrogenic foods that lower thyroid function include peanuts, peanut butter, and millet.

Polyunsaturated oils. These oils include soy, corn, safflower, sunflower, and cottonseed. They interfere with thyroid gland function and the response of tissues to thyroid hormone because these longer-chain fatty acids are deposited in cells more often as rancid, oxidized fat. Oxidized oils block thyroid hormone secretions. This impairs the body's ability to convert T4 to T3, which creates the enzymes needed to convert fats to energy. When this breakdown occurs, one can develop symptoms typical of hypothyroidism.

Food allergens

When it comes to food-related allergies that impact the thyroid gland, it is not like eating a nut or a shrimp and getting an immediate reaction. The type of reaction that disrupts thyroid function is a delayed interaction with food antigens that can occur up to four days after eating the food. The two most prevalent food-related reactions come from dairy and wheat. These two foods are known in alternative medicine to be highly correlated with autoimmune thyroiditis. Dairy and wheat gluten are often removed from diets of thyroid patients with good success. The *Journal of Clinical Gastroenterology* demonstrated that those allergic to gluten had a much greater risk of thyroid abnormalities.[15]

Iodized salt

Replace iodized salt with Celtic sea salt because table salt is a problem for some people with thyroid challenges. Also, choose only natural sources of iodine.

Halogens: chlorine, fluoride, and bromine

Halogens (fluorine, chlorine, bromine, and astatine) are now becoming ubiquitous in our environment and have major consequences for thyroid function. Since iodine shares chemical properties with other halogens like chlorine, fluorine, and bromine, these halogens can displace iodine and disrupt thyroid function. Chlorine is added to our municipal water supply. Fluoride is also added to our water as well as toothpastes and is used in dental treatments. Many popular sports and electrolyte drinks contain brominated vegetable oil. Bromine also is used in some baked goods and fire-retardant compounds. Bromine-based fire retardants used in carpets, mattresses, upholstery, furniture, and various electronic equipment have become suspect for causing or contributing to hypothyroidism.[16]

A study published in *Physiological Research* showed that bromine intake blocks iodine uptake by the thyroid and increases its excretion through the urine.[17] Bromism, a condition of excess bromine intake, is known to have drastic effects on the nervous system—a situation common among low-thyroid sufferers. Based on research, bromides have also been linked to behavioral problems, neurodevelopmental delays, and attention-deficit hyperactivity disorder (ADD/ADHD) in children.

Splenda (sucralose) is made when hydroxyl groups in a sugar molecule are replaced with chlorine molecules—the same chlorine atoms used to disinfect swimming pools. We know that polychlorinated biphenyls and organochlorines from pesticides and other sources alter thyroid function and impede weight loss. The journal *Obesity Reviews* highlighted the effect chlorine molecules have on thyroid and weight loss. This article showed that chlorine molecules that accumulated in human fat tissue are released during weight loss and impair thyroid function, potentially leading to weight-loss resistance.[18] The fact that Splenda, which contains artificially placed chlorine molecules, is marketed as a "diet sweetener" seems to be an oxymoron of advertising, based on this research.

But thyroid problems and weight-loss resistance are not the only concerns with this product. We do not know the long-term health effects that Splenda will have on the human body because it's a relatively new product, but the Food and Drug Administration (FDA) has given a review of possible side-effects from consuming this artificial sweetener, including enlarged liver and kidneys, decreased white blood cell count, reduced growth rate, and decreased fetal body weight.[19] I recommend that you completely avoid this sweetener.

Mercury

Mercury is a toxic metal that can significantly impact the thyroid. There is ample evidence that mercury leaches from dental amalgam fillings and contributes to thyroid disease and anemia along with a host of other physical problems. While large doses of mercury can induce hyperthyroidism, smaller amounts can induce hypothyroidism by interfering with both the production of thyroxine (T4) and the conversion of T4 to T3. Mercury also disturbs the metabolism of copper and zinc, which are two minerals critical to thyroid function. Gray hair can be an indication of mercury accumulation, more so in women than men.

Mercury can cause disruptions to the immune system and promotes the production of antibodies produced by the immune system, which also are involved in autoimmune thyroid disease. There are different forms of mercury—organic and inorganic—that can have different effects on the thyroid. It is believed that estrogen and milk can cause an increase in the absorption of mercury. Mercury also hinders the availability of selenium-dependant enzymes. These are the same enzymes used by the thyroid to make thyroid hormone.

Radiation

It is known that radiation exposure increases the risk for thyroid cancer. Environmental exposure, such as that from nuclear power plants and radioactive fallout, and exposure from medical procedures are problematic. Airport scanners pose more of a problem for developing skin cancer. The risk of thyroid disease from radiation exposure increases in individuals who are iodine deficient. When you supplement your diet with iodine, it is taken up by the thyroid gland, which then blocks radiation uptake into the thyroid, reducing your risk for thyroid cancer—an epidemic in the United States likely due in part to excess CT scans combined with iodine deficiency. Potassium iodide is used to treat radiation emergency caused by exposure to radioactive iodides, but excess iodine can be harmful to health. However, water-soluble iodine seems to be much less problematic. It's best to increase your iodine intake with food such as kelp powder, dulse, sea vegetables, sea food, and cranberries (all iodine rich) because radioactive iodine will drop into iodine receptor cites that have no iodine in them as a result of iodine deficiencies.

It's also important to increase your antioxidant intake. Radiation within the body generates massive amounts of damaging free radicals that can harm your DNA, which can lead to cancer a decade or two later. Therefore it's imperative to maximize your overall antioxidant intake by juicing and eating plenty of vegetables, especially the dark leafy greens, along with taking extra vitamins C and E, selenium, N-acetyl cysteine, alpha-lipoic acid, and coenzyme Q_{10}. Unfortunately the antioxidant defense system of many Americans is in poor condition. Spirulina and chlorella are antioxidant rich and were used extensively by the Russians after the Chernobyl nuclear plant disaster. Miso is also protective and helpful when exposed to radiation. It was used in Japan after World War II. Following the Nagasaki bombing, a group of macrobiotic doctors and their patients avoided radiation sickness and did not get leukemia by eating brown rice, miso, and seaweed.[20]

Juice more chlorophyll-rich foods such as wheatgrass, barley grass, kale, collard greens, beet greens, Swiss chard, parsley, rapini, kohlrabi leaves, and dandelion leaves, which help to strengthen cells, transport oxygen, and detoxify the blood and liver, helping to bind up polluting elements and stimulate RNA production. (I recommend juicing them because you can consume much more by juicing than just eating the plants.) Also, eat and juice more sulfur-containing vegetables, including broccoli, cabbage, mustard greens, and garlic, which combine with heavy metals and prevent free-radical damage. Cilantro helps to remove heavy metals and radioactive materials from the brain. Juice up a large handful of cilantro each day.

Take baths with baking soda and magnesium salts. Uranium will bond with sodium bicarbonate (baking soda). This will help to protect the kidneys and cleanse the body. To combat radioactive fallout or exposure to radiation, start by using one pound of baking soda in a bath; add to that magnesium in the form of bath flakes, Dead Sea salt, or Epsom salts.

Other substances

Caffeine and alcohol. It's important to avoid coffee, black tea, green tea, sodas, chocolate, and all alcoholic beverages.

Vaccines. Thimerosal is the mercury-containing preservative used in many vaccines. It has also been used in contact lens solutions, eye drops, and immunoglobulins. Additionally, it is used in patch testing for people who have dermatitis, conjunctivitis, and other potentially allergic reactions. The body uses selenium to stabilize mercury in the body and keep it from doing damage. Similar to the story with halogens and iodine, mercury uses up this valuable nutrient, as well as causing various other problems.

Electromagnetic fields (EMFs). EMFs are everywhere in our modern world—microwave, cell phone, alarm clock, computer, electrical cables, and the list goes on and on. They all emit electromagnetic waves, which are known to penetrate and influence the body. The thyroid may be among the most sensitive organs to EMF radiation. The July 2005 *Toxicology Letters* show just how sensitive the thyroid is to EMF. In this study, researchers looked at the effect of the equivalent EMF dose delivered by a cell phone. The researchers wanted to see how this level of EMF impacted thyroid function. T3, T4, and thyroid-stimulating hormone (TSH) were all decreased a significant degree under the influence of the EMFs.[21]

THE LINK BETWEEN ADRENAL FATIGUE AND THYROID CONDITIONS

Of the millions of people who are diagnosed with thyroid conditions, many of them also have or develop adrenal fatigue. Adrenal fatigue is a collection of symptoms that results when the adrenal glands do not function at their optimal level. The fatigue is not relieved by sleep. As a result, changes may occur in carbohydrate, protein, and fat metabolism; blood sugar balance; energy production; fluid and electrolyte balance; cardiovascular function; sleep patterns; mood; menstrual and menopausal symptoms; and even sex drive. People whose adrenals are fatigued often have to use coffee, colas, and other stimulants to get going in the morning and to prop themselves up during the day.

Symptoms of Adrenal Fatigue

- Extremely tired, especially in the morning
- Have trouble getting up, even when you've had enough sleep
- Find it difficult to obtain quality sleep
- Crave sweet and salty foods
- Feel stressed out most of the time
- Feel rundown or overwhelmed
- Have trouble bouncing back from an illness or stressful situation
- Decreased sex drive

- Feel more awake, alert, and energetic after 6:00 p.m. than you do all day

MANY THYROID CONDITIONS ARE DUE TO ADRENAL GLAND PROBLEMS

It's important to understand that in many cases a malfunctioning thyroid gland isn't the actual cause of the hypothyroid condition. Other areas of the body may be responsible, and while different areas of the body can be affected, in many cases it's weakened adrenal glands that lead to the development of low thyroid function.

If a health care professional aims treatment only at the thyroid gland and ignores the adrenals and other areas and factors, there may not be a chance of restoring thyroid or adrenal function back to normal. Just prescribing thyroid medication for the rest of a person's life (or radioactive iodine for those with hyperthyroidism) will not address the root problem. The entire endocrine system, including the adrenal glands, needs to be evaluated.

WHAT CAUSES ADRENAL FATIGUE?

Adrenal fatigue often develops over a period of years due to unhealthy lifestyle factors such as poor eating habits, poor sleep patterns, and/or chronic stress. For example, someone who eats a lot of refined foods and sugar will have an imbalance in the hormones insulin and cortisol. Eating poorly can, over time, lead to insulin resistance and eventually diabetes, which usually takes years to develop. The constant secretion of cortisol in response to eating poorly and/or dealing with chronic stress can weaken the adrenal glands and eventually lead to adrenal fatigue.

Similarly, not getting enough sleep can weaken the adrenals. Many people stay up late watching television, surfing the Internet, staying out with friends, or studying. They get only five to seven hours of sleep; some even less. This is not enough. Most people need eight hours of sleep; some even more. An occasional short night of sleep is not a problem, but on a regular basis, it can affect cortisol levels and weaken adrenal glands. And not dealing with stress effectively has a similar effect on the adrenal and thyroid glands, weakening both.

Trauma, which can be either physical or emotional in nature, such as a car accident, the death of a loved one, a divorce, or loss of a job, can trigger this disorder as well. This doesn't mean that such traumas cause the immediate development of adrenal fatigue, but they can be the trigger that over time leads to its development.

When the adrenal glands are weakened, it puts the body in a state of catabolism—the body begins breaking down. When the body is in a catabolic state, the thyroid gland will slow down (become hypothyroid) in an attempt to conserve energy and prevent the body from breaking down more. This makes sense in that hypothyroidism slows down the metabolism.

There is no magic bullet or supplement that can quickly cure these conditions. But by changing your lifestyle, you can heal these glands and restore your health. It usually doesn't take too long before you start feeling better, and symptoms should lessen within a few weeks if you strictly adhere to the Juice Lady's living foods program. It will take time, though, to completely heal. It's very important to remember that when you start feeling a little better, you should not abandon your healthy lifestyle program.

Adrenal Fatigue Followed My Attack

If you read the introduction, you know that I was attacked in the night by a burglar while I was house sitting for friends. Following the attack, I suffered extreme adrenal fatigue. I was so tired I could barely drag myself through a day. It felt like I had a ball and chain wrapped around my body. Just getting dressed in the morning was a huge effort. I remember sitting on the floor in the corner of my bedroom thinking that I was so tired I couldn't get up off the floor. Life was so painful and difficult that it didn't seem worth it to go on. I remember thinking I could go deep inside my soul where there was peace and hide. But I recalled something about a catatonic state (one of near unconsciousness often brought on by shock) from psychology 101. My professor had mentioned that it was hard to bring people out of that state. I thought I'd better not go there just in case I would not want to be there some day. I decided to hang on for just one more day, albeit by a thin thread of hope that things might improve. Obviously, they did.

I looked at my picture on my website the other day. It didn't seem possible that the glowing person I was looking at was the same person who once sat in that room one thought away from "checking out" for good.

Healing the adrenals, indeed the entire body, takes work. It takes the best nutrition you can possibly eat and drink, with a lot of that being live foods rich in biophotons that give life to your body. It takes nutritional supplements of superior quality. It may take a few IVs of Meyer's Cocktail (vitamin C drip with other nutrients), which is what I got, along with prayer and intense emotional work.

You can restore burned-out adrenals that are so exhausted they're barely producing cortisol. You can heal your body that feels too tired to move. I know you can. If I could do it, so can you. We're not all that different, you and I. So go for it! Give it all you have. One day, my friend, you'll be standing in your dream as well, just as I'm standing in mine.

THE LIVING FOODS REVOLUTION FOR STRESSED ADRENALS AND THYROID

Sample diet plan (Day 1)

Upon rising
Start your day with ⅛ to ½ teaspoon of Celtic sea salt or kelp powder dissolved in a glass of water, juice, or herbal tea. Drink another glass at your lowest energy point during the day. When the adrenal glands are fatigued, they do not produce enough aldosterone. Aldosterone regulates the amount of sodium and potassium in the body. When aldosterone becomes deficient, not enough salt is retained in the body. Have you been craving salt? This is probably the reason.

Avoid caffeine
Coffee, black tea, and possibly even green tea for a while (although it has ⅓ the caffeine of coffee) should be avoided. Even white tea, which has the least caffeine of all, may be too much for your weak adrenals. Pushing your adrenals with caffeine is like whipping a tired horse that needs to rest.

Breakfast
Try the Adrenal Booster Cocktail (page 180) followed by a Healthy Green Smoothie (page 190).

Midmorning or midafternoon
Have a fresh juice midmorning and/or mid- to late afternoon. Dark green juices are particularly beneficial.

Lunch and dinner
Raw foods are helpful as well for their superior nutrients and biophotons. You can choose raw food recipes, some cooked food recipes, and some animal products that are organic, grass fed, and free range, if you are not vegan. Eat lots of high-fiber vegetables. There is a need for high-quality protein as well. You may need some animal protein for a while unless you

go mostly raw and really focus on getting enough high-quality protein from seeds, nuts, sprouts, and dark leafy greens. You may also need to supplement with free-form amino acids. The amino acid program has made a significant difference for many people that I've worked with. (If you suspect you have adrenal fatigue, you may want to take the Adrenal Saliva Test. See Appendix A.) Also, keep your blood sugar balanced. Eat smaller meals and a couple of very nutritious snacks during the day.

Nutrients and juices (daily recommendations)

Vitamin C
2,000–4,000 mg/day with bioflavonoids
Foods to juice: hot peppers, kale, parsley, collard, turnip greens, broccoli, mustard greens, watercress, lemons with white part, and spinach

Vitamin E
800 IU/day with mixed tocopherols
Foods to juice: spinach, asparagus, and carrots

Niacin
125–150 mg/day, as niacinamide

Pyridoxine (vitamin B_6)
150 mg/day
Foods to juice: spinach, kale, avocado (green smoothies)

Pantothenic acid (vitamin B_5)
1,200–1,500 mg/day
Foods to juice: broccoli, kale

Vitamin B-100 Complex
I suggest B Complex 12 by Thorne; take as directed.

Magnesium citrate
400–1,200 mg/day
Foods to juice: beet greens, spinach, parsley, dandelion greens, garlic, beets, carrots, celery, avocado (green smoothies)

Trace minerals
Multi-minerals; they have a calming effect
I suggest Citramins (multi-minerals) by Thorne; take as directed.
Foods to juice: Dark leafy greens are especially rich in minerals.

Herbs

Rhodiola rosea
Enhances memory and concentration; has been shown to reduce stress-induced fatigue and improve mental performance

Holy basil leaf
Helps to normalize cortisol in times of stress

Wild oats milky seed
Supports the nervous system

Schisandra berry
Helps with energy, endurance, and resistance to stress

Ashwagandha
Has been shown to have a sedating effect on the body and helps to rebuild the digestive and nervous system

Siberian ginseng
Has been used traditionally to stimulate and nourish the adrenal glands and increases mental alertness

Cordyceps
A Chinese mushroom used for supporting the adrenal gland; can also help the immune function

Licorice root (not the candy)
Provides a lift for the adrenal glands and improves resistance to stress; should be used in small amounts according to directions since it can raise blood pressure in higher quantities

Lifestyle Factors That May Contribute to Adrenal Fatigue

- Lack of sleep
- Poor food choices (white flour, low fiber, sugar, too few vegetables and fruit, lack of raw food)
- Using sweet or salty food and sweetened or caffeinated drinks as stimulants when tired
- Staying up late even though tired
- Feeling or acting powerless
- Continually driving yourself
- Striving to be perfect
- Staying in double binds—no-win situations

- Too few enjoyable and rejuvenating activities
- Trauma, loss, shock, extreme disappointment

LIFESTYLE CHANGES THAT HELP ADRENAL FATIGUE

Reduce stressors. This is a most important step. Emotional stressors such as marital, family, friend, or financial problems need to be dealt with and responded to in a healthy way. Stress causes the adrenal glands to produce more cortisol, which deposits weight on the belly. When the adrenal glands become exhausted, however, they produce less and less cortisol.

Sleep. Rest and sleep are extremely important to heal the adrenals. Get eight to nine hours of sleep or more. Also rest after meals and at midmorning and midafternoon if possible. Adrenal fatigue is a common cause of insomnia. There are two types of insomnia: adrenal hyper function (inability to fall asleep) and adrenal fatigue (inability to stay asleep). If you have hyper-adrenal function, you may have higher than normal levels of cortisol at bedtime so you can't fall asleep. If you can't stay asleep, you may have very low levels of cortisol and may be getting too much neurotransmitter stimulation. As blood sugar levels start to drop during the middle of the night, normally your adrenal glands are secreting cortisol to help push your blood sugar levels back up. That is normal and is what's supposed to happen. If your glands cannot produce enough cortisol to keep your blood sugar levels balanced, you will shift to a backup system that involves the release of epinephrine and norepinephrine. These hormones are central nervous system stimulants that will wake you up. This is why you may seem to be wide-awake with a racing mind around the same time every night, such as 2:00, 3:00, or 4:00 a.m.

Sleep medications are not the answer. They have many side effects and don't cure the problem. (See Appendix A for the amino acid program that helps balance brain neurotransmitters so you can start sleeping deeply all night.)

Gentle exercise is beneficial, but vigorous exercise depletes the adrenals. Deep breathing and stretching are very beneficial.

Detoxification. Using an infrared sauna will greatly speed up recovery. If you are in adrenal burnout, use the sauna daily for no more than thirty minutes. Once or twice a week is excellent for maintenance.

Chapter 5

Living Foods for Detoxification

Your body is a temple, but only if you treat it as one.
—Astrid Alauda

THINK ABOUT YOUR body as you would your car. What if you never changed your oil or filters in your car? It's the same thing with your body. To keep it humming along like a well-maintained vehicle, you need to periodically cleanse the blood and its filter systems, which are your organs of elimination.

Because of all the pollution in our world and our occasional, or maybe constant, unwise food choices, our normal body processes can get overwhelmed. Toxic substances, mucus, and congestion get trapped in our tissues and tissue spaces. Our body attempts to protect us by enclosing toxins in mucus and fat cells, and it will hang onto those fat cells to save us. We may not be able to lose weight unless we cleanse our body first. The same goes for getting well and achieving vibrant health.

It's estimated that the average adult has between 5 and 10 pounds of accumulated toxic waste in their cells, tissues, and organs, particularly the colon. (That's 5 to 10 pounds we could really feel great about dropping!) Toxic substances that accumulate throughout the body can weaken and congest our organs and systems of elimination and lead to diseases such as cancer. They also mess up our weight-loss goals. If we go on a very strict diet that forces the body to let go of fat cells for survival, the weight will come right back on when we stop the program.

Toxins come from a number of sources such as the environment, unhealthy food choices, and internal by-products of metabolism, called endotoxins. This toxic soup mix consists of chemicals, pesticides, drug residues, heavy metals, and food additives, along with by-products from digestion as well as yeasts, fungus, and parasites. This stuff can pile up inside the body like gunk inside home plumbing. If they are not broken down and eliminated, they get stored throughout the body. The body especially likes to store them in fat cells; it's one of the safest places to place them. It will even make more of these little storage units as needed. They also jam up the works in organs like the liver and kidneys. They can be found in the large and small intestines. And they hide in the mucous lining of the lungs and sinuses. Additionally, toxins are distributed into the cells and tissues of the brain where they can cause a lot of cognitive and emotional problems like brain fog and emotional outbursts. And they get deposited in the skin and bones as well.

Toxins make us sick, weak, overweight, and unable to fight off infections, and they cause pain in our muscles and joints. Toxic molecules, known as free radicals, damage our cells, creating numerous health problems, and accelerate aging. This is why it's so crucial to periodically cleanse the body.

With more than 87,000 chemicals used in commerce,[1] we are exposed to thousands of toxins on a daily basis! Where do they go? More importantly, how do we get rid of them? *The Juice Lady's Living Foods Revolution* will help you begin the process of cleansing. You can join the thousands of people who testify to the fact that pain is gone, weight has melted away, and many health challenges have cleared up when they cleansed their body.

Study Shows Pregnant Women Have Harmful Toxins in Their Bodies

The University of California–San Francisco (UCSF) conducted a study revealing that virtually every single pregnant woman in the United States carries multiple harmful environmental chemicals in her body, even some that have been banned for years. This information is not a big shock because it's common knowledge that we're all exposed to multiple environmental chemicals. However, this was the first study of its kind to focus on the environmental chemical burden of pregnant women in particular.[2]

This study makes a good case for encouraging all women who want to get pregnant to first complete a total-body cleansing program. Toxins can contribute to birth defects and illnesses in babies.

When the organs and systems of elimination get behind in their work, the toxic sludge backs up into all the supporting systems just as dirty water backs up in a stopped-up sink. First the intestines build up mucus and putrefaction, causing nutrients to not be properly absorbed. Poisons are absorbed back into the bloodstream. The liver becomes overwhelmed and congested, stones may form, and the blood is not purified properly, so more toxins build up in the bloodstream. The filtration system in the kidneys works hard to excrete toxic-laden urine, but it can become overwhelmed too, and some waste can get recirculated. The skin is the largest organ of elimination, and it may show signs of toxicity such as rashes, pimples, acne, or other skin conditions when it can't deal with excess waste.

This downward spiral continues affecting more than just the elimination system. Toxins are shunted off to storage in fat cells so our delicate tissues and organs will be protected from the acidity (toxins are acidic). The body holds on to fat as a protective measure. Consequently, we have difficulty losing weight. These acidic pollutants collect in cells, tissues, organs, and the fluids between the cells, making cellular metabolism inefficient at best. They can show up as cellulite—the stuff that sticks on our thighs like a glob of cottage cheese. And they can clog our sinuses, lungs, and the passages of the lymphatic system. The result of this toxic overload is sickness, tiredness, pain, weight gain, and eventually disease.

Cleansing for Weight Loss

My roommate went on the weekend cleanse to detoxify her body and lost 5 pounds, adding to her loss of 10 pounds in just two weeks. I haven't lost any weight yet, but I have more energy and I feel great. My kids love it too!

—Victoria (from *Juicing, Fasting and Detoxing for Life*'s Amazon page)

FLUSH AWAY THAT LUMPY SKIN!

It's not just another fat. Cellulite is that lumpy, bumpy orange-peel-looking stuff that consists of irregular fat deposits. Essentially, this fat is trapped within connective tissues, and the affected areas are full of fluid, toxins, lymph, and waste. Most of us aren't too happy about these particular dimples. They are usually found on the thighs, hips, and buttocks. Frustratingly, many dieters find that no matter how hard they work at exercise and strict dieting, this stuff sticks to the thighs like caramel on an apple—even when they've dropped down a size or two.

Because it's quite different from your garden-variety kind of pudgy fat, cellulite has to be tackled uniquely. It is associated with poorly functioning blood vessels, constipation, poor lymphatic drainage, and toxicity. If blood vessels are weak and sluggish, fluids and toxins will accumulate quickly, making it difficult for the body to burn fat in the affected areas.

Constipation contributes to cellulite because poor elimination causes wastes and toxins to remain in the body rather than being purged out. It's then absorbed back into the system. A sluggish, poorly functioning colon means that toxic wastes are also affecting the efficiency of organs such as the liver and kidneys. And since the lymphatic system has no pump, there's only one way to move that garbage-laden fluid through the body— and that's exercise and/or lymphatic drainage massage. One of the best buys you could make in this respect is the lymphasizer, which gets your lymph moving. (See Appendix A.)

Consuming sugar, refined salt (sodium chloride), caffeine, alcohol, tobacco, unhealthy fats and oils, and refined carbohydrates, taxes your lymphatic and circulatory systems. This makes it much harder for your body to eliminate waste—and far easier for fat to get stored as cellulite. Some experts believe it is toxins that cause this fat to become trapped in the first place and held in these lumpy spots.

This kind of fat can't be eradicated just by eating healthy foods or by exercise. Nor can it be cured with topical treatments. Though creams, lotions, or massage may help a bit, they will not wipe away the lumps. You can rub, massage, and wrap this fat in seaweed every day of your life, but this stuff is not going to disappear unless you internally cleanse your body (especially your colon and liver), improve your circulation and metabolism, get your lymph moving, and nourish your body with living foods and juices. Also, as you boost your metabolism, the circulatory and lymphatic systems will work better, and you'll increase your chances of evicting the bulges and bumps.

Changing your diet and detoxifying your body are your passport to smooth skin. I know firsthand that this works. You have to flush out the toxins, plain and simple, if you want to be cellulite free. It's also important to nourish and condition the areas affected with cellulite in order to strengthen blood vessels and tissues and step up circulation. When toxins are removed and blood vessels and surrounding tissues are nourished, then it is possible for the fat to be used as energy. That's when you see this stuff start to disappear. Your thighs don't have to look like a pitted golf ball any longer. You can be trimmer and sleeker because of your cleansing program.

Studies Reveal Pesticides and Other Toxins Make Us Fat

Researchers showed that the common herbicide atrazine causes sex changes in fish, and it also makes rats fat regardless of their feeding behavior. "It's possible that the sorts of genes that play a role in reading signals on the way from the brain to the periphery to regulate fat are being acted upon by pesticides and...things that are in the environment," said Kaveh Ashrafi, MD, PhD.

Dr. Ashrafi mentioned another study in which mice were exposed for five days to diethylstilbestrol (DES)—used in feed for factory-farm livestock and poultry—while in utero. The mice had normal birth weights and normal growth rates, but they ended up much fatter over time even though they had the same eating and activity habits as mice that were not exposed to DES.

Could drug residues in commercial meat be contributing to weight gain for people who eat commercial animal products frequently? Dr. Ashrafi said, "Maybe environmental toxins are essentially drugs that we are taking without knowing it, and they're acting in this process to promote fat regulation."[3]

How Toxic Are You?

Do you have symptoms of toxicity? Take the toxicity quiz below, and give yourself a point for every symptom that describes you. If you score even a few points on the quiz, I recommend that you go through my detox programs. But even if you don't score any points, everyone should detox their body at least once a year. It's like changing your vehicle's oil every three thousand miles or every three months, whichever comes first. You don't wait until your car starts having problems to change your oil. You do this to keep it "symptom free." As you cleanse each organ of elimination, you'll improve your health, become stronger, look younger, and remain symptom free.

The Toxicity Quiz

- ❏ Aches and pains
- ❏ Acid reflux
- ❏ Arthritis
- ❏ Bloating and gas
- ❏ Cellulite
- ❏ Constipation
- ❏ Dizziness
- ❏ Emotional and mental problems
- ❏ Headaches
- ❏ Hormone imbalances
- ❏ Inability to lose weight
- ❏ Indigestion
- ❏ Irritability

- ❏ Lack of energy and fatigue
- ❏ Overweight
- ❏ Premature aging
- ❏ Restlessness
- ❏ Sinus problems
- ❏ Skin problems
- ❏ Stressful feelings
- ❏ Trouble sleeping/insomnia
- ❏ Visual problems
- ❏ Weakness

One of the initial benefits you should notice after you've cleansed your body is that you have more energy. When your system is overburdened with waste, congestion, and toxins, a lot of energy is used to deal with that just to keep you going. Once the toxins are removed, your body doesn't need to work as hard, and you experience more energy.

The Living Foods Revolution Begins With the Detoxification Process

By embarking on the living foods program, you will begin the detoxification process. Raw juices and live foods are chock-full of antioxidants, which bind to toxins and carry them out of the body. Antioxidants latch onto the "bad guys" like Pac-Man eating every dot or power pellet.

A number of people have contacted me with symptoms associated with detoxification not long after beginning the living foods and juicing program. It's important to know what symptoms might be part of the cleansing process.

Cleansing Reactions

Cleansing reactions, also known as the Herxheimer reaction or healing crisis, is believed to be a reaction caused by organisms dying off and toxins being released into the body faster than the body may comfortably handle. Usually these symptoms last only a short time. Drink plenty of water and fresh vegetable juice to flush the system. Also, enemas help release toxins quickly from the colon and can relieve symptoms, which include the following:

- Bad breath
- Bloating
- Chills, cold extremities

- Constipation or diarrhea
- Elevated heart rate
- Fatigue
- Fever (usually low grade)
- Flu-like symptoms
- Headache
- Hives and rash (sometimes assumed to be an allergic reaction)
- Hypotension (low blood pressure)
- Increased joint or muscle pain
- Itching, scratching
- Nausea
- Swollen glands
- Unusual perspiration

If you experience some of these reactions, drink more water. Flush your colon with a colonic or enema. And you'll need to do more work on specific organs of elimination if you want to truly remove the toxic waste that has accumulated over the years. After you complete various organ cleanses, your energy and vitality will be renewed, and you'll lose fat and cellulite. You should notice that stubborn symptoms disappear, and ailments or illnesses will lessen or disappear. You should also experience the glow of health and vitality that may have been eluding you for years.

We have built-in processes for dealing with toxins, poisons, chemicals, yeasts, parasites, and internal by-products of metabolism. But there's so much toxic stuff in our world that we need to do extra cleansing to support our organs of elimination.

Benefits of Detoxification

- Better health
- Better sleep
- Digestive system cleared of mucus and congestion
- Fewer mood swings
- Greater sense of well-being
- Improved digestion
- Improved skin and younger appearance
- Increased mental clarity
- Lessening or disappearance of pain
- More creativity

- Purified blood
- Re-colonization of healthy bacteria
- Reduced cravings for sugar, salt, junk foods, alcohol, and nicotine
- Renewed joy
- Renewed vitality
- Stronger immune system
- Weight loss

SPECIFIC CLEANSE PROGRAMS

Completing specific detox programs will help you remove the causes of disease, aging, and weight gain. It can help you heal, if you're ill, and restore your health and vitality. Specific cleanses will give your organs, blood, and systems of elimination a true "spring cleaning."

SAUNA DETOX

One of the best ways to get rid of toxins, and especially plastic toxins (some say the only way to get rid of plastic toxins), is using a sauna. It is important to sweat to cleanse toxins out of the body. Sweat is one of the best ways to eliminate fat-soluble toxins, including perfluorocarbons (PFCs), and can help protect you from the accumulation of most of these vandals.

Toxic chemicals and metals can be removed faster with a sauna than with any other method. Repeated use of the sauna slowly restores skin elimination that has been clogged by a host of waste products.

There are two types of saunas—traditional wood, electric, or gas fired, and infrared. The traditional sauna requires preheating, and the intense heat is difficult for many people to tolerate. The infrared sauna uses ceramic heating elements and does not require preheating. It heats the body while the air remains cool. Sweating begins more quickly and cellular elimination is promoted more effectively than when using other saunas.

The Sauna Detoxification Steps

- Spend no more than thirty minutes at a time in the sauna with a ten-minute break, if you return to the sauna.
- The temperature should not exceed 110 degrees.

- Drink a 16-ounce glass of fresh vegetable juice or mineralized water before entering the sauna.
- Ventilate the sauna whenever you use it, which may be built into the design, to avoid breathing toxic gases your body releases.
- After the sauna, drink a glass of purified water.
- Take a warm or cool, not hot, shower. Do not use soap, which leaves a film that clogs the pores. Use a bath brush or loofa to wash off sweat and dead skin cells. Include your face and hair, as well. Don't use traditional shampoo and hair rinse that are loaded with chemicals. Use only a natural organic shampoo and conditioner. Avoid creams and lotions afterward. You can use organic coconut oil on your skin.
- Sit or lie down for at least ten minutes afterward.
- Add extra Celtic sea salt or kelp granules to your diet to replace minerals lost through sweating, or take a packet of Emergen-C.
- Eat only organic, whole foods grown on mineral-rich soil.
- Always make sure you get plenty of rest while detoxing, and get at least eight hours of sleep.
- Get at least thirty minutes of gentle exercise each day, such as walking.
- Deeply breathe in clean, fresh air.
- Avoid all toxic chemicals.
- Keep a positive attitude. A proverb says that a merry heart is good medicine.

THE INTESTINAL CLEANSE

When we consume processed food; excessively cooked food; fried food; junk food; spoiled food; refined carbs; sweets like candy, chocolate, cookies, and ice cream; coffee; sodas; sports drinks; alcohol; and prescription or recreational drugs, we can stimulate mucous secretions throughout our entire alimentary canal. This is normal; it's the body's natural way of protecting itself against an occasional encounter with spoiled or irritating food. But when we consume these substances every day, and for some people almost every meal, mucus and waste build up on the intestinal wall just as filth builds up in the bathroom pipes. Pancreatic juices help to digest food and cleanse mucus from the intestines. But continual poor food choices lead to constant mucous secretion, and the digestive juices cannot break down and eliminate this large overload of waste.

Mucous and waste buildup can interfere with nutrient absorption because it forms a hard, rubbery kind of layer in the intestinal tract. I was skeptical about this until I tried an intestinal cleanse program. Then I saw firsthand the truth of what I'd read.

Many of our nutrients are absorbed through the small intestine. If it's coated with this rubbery type of plaque, we're not going to absorb a significant portion of the nutrients we eat. Also, this mucous and waste buildup provides a hiding place and breeding ground for *Candida albicans* and parasites. I struggled with parasites and candidiasis for years, until I discovered the effectiveness of intestinal detoxification.

As intestinal waste builds up, motility becomes less effective and food takes longer to pass through the digestive tract, which is called constipation. The longer the "transit time," the longer the toxic waste matter sits in the bowel, which allows it to putrefy, ferment forming gases, and possibly be reabsorbed. The longer your body is exposed to putrefying food in your intestines, the greater the risk of developing diseases. Even with one bowel movement per day, you will still have at least three meals worth of waste decaying in your colon at all times.

Disease usually begins with a toxic bowel. Infrequent or poor quality bowel movements over an extended period of time may be very destructive to your health. Those having fewer bowel movements than one a day are harboring a potentially fertile breeding ground for serious diseases such as colon cancer.

As you transition to the living foods lifestyle program, which is rich in raw fruits and vegetables, with a smaller percentage of cooked foods and little or no processed foods, you'll be helping to keep your digestive system free of mucoid plaque. Regular and easy elimination will be the norm for you (stool softeners won't be needed), toxins will not build up, and your digestion will improve.

It's not hard to see why a clean intestinal tract is so important to good health. An intestinal cleanse program will help you reduce waste buildup in the intestinal tract and allow for more efficient absorption of nutrients. If you have an intestinal disease, such as Crohn's disease or diverticulitis, check with a holistic doctor before beginning.

Intestinal Cleanse Plan: Supporting Foods and Herbs

You should cleanse your colon for at least one week before doing other cleanses. But if you have never done a colon cleanse before, you may need to do several weeks of cleansing to clear out the plaque.

- Follow the living foods vegan menu plan, selecting a large percentage of raw foods while cleansing your colon. If your digestion is strong, you can eat all raw. If your digestion needs some help, then eat raw in the morning and at noon, and some lightly cooked vegetables in the evening. Avoid grains, unless they are sprouted, as this will slow your cleansing. And all animal products should be avoided, as this will stop the cleansing process.

- You may choose to go on a one- to three-day vegetable juice fast. This will greatly facilitate the colon cleanse process.

- Drink at least eight glasses of purified water each day.

- Start your day with a cup of hot water and the juice of one quarter of a lemon with a dash of cayenne pepper. This will have a bit of a laxative effect, stimulate digestive juices, and get your liver moving.

- In the morning and before bed, mix 1 tablespoon of bentonite clay in a glass of water. Bentonite is a type of edible clay that acts as a bulk laxative by absorbing water to form a gel. It binds toxins such as pesticides and helps to carry them out of the colon. Add 1 tablespoon of ground flaxseeds (or psyllium powder or fiber blend that's premade) mixed well with the bentonite clay and water; drink right away because it gels and will become too thick to drink if you wait. This will absorb water and expand in the colon, and it helps to remove toxins and mucus.

- Wait at least thirty minutes before eating.

- Before bed, take an herbal cleansing product that contains such ingredients as cascara sagrada, Chinese rhubarb root, barberry root, dandelion root, fringetree root bark, aronia fruit, chebulic and belleric myrobalan fruit, meadowsweet aerial plant, English plantain, ginger root, fennel seed, peppermint leaf, fenugreek seed, and licorice root.

- Take probiotics to replenish the good bacteria in the colon.

- Take enemas or colonics to assist in eliminating wastes

NOTE: If you take medication, bentonite clay should be reduced and taken away from medication as it may interfere with absorption.

For intestinal cleanse products that have all the ingredients in the best formulation, see Appendix A.

KIDNEY CLEANSE

The kidneys perform many important functions, including:

- Elimination of wastes
- Excretion of urine
- Blood pressure regulation
- Balancing pH—acid/alkaline balance
- Balancing fluid and electrolytes

Poor dietary habits such as eating refined carbohydrates (sweets and white flour products such as baked goods), drinking too much alcohol, eating too much animal protein and fat, consuming mucus-forming foods such as dairy products, and eating too much refined salt, along with taking prescription drugs, eating food sprayed with pesticides, and contamination with mercury, radiation, and environmental toxins—all can overload the kidneys, making them less effective at eliminating waste. This reduced efficiency contributes to more congestion in the body, kidney stone development, and other kidney and bladder ailments.

Symptoms of Kidney Congestion or Toxicity

Check off the box next to any symptoms you are experiencing. If you have even a few of these symptoms, I recommend a kidney cleanse.

- ❑ Blood in the urine
- ❑ Burning or pain during urination
- ❑ Cloudy urine
- ❑ Cold sensation in the lower half of the body
- ❑ Dark circles under the eyes
- ❑ Frequent urination (especially at night)
- ❑ Foul-smelling or dark urine
- ❑ Incontinence
- ❑ Pain in or around the eyes

Cleansing juices and teas for the kidneys

Choose one or more these teas:

Watermelon seed tea. At least once a day for three days, drink watermelon seed tea. Prepare it by pouring a pint of boiling water over a tablespoonful of ground or chopped watermelon seeds and allowing it to steep. Let it cool a bit, then strain and drink. If possible, the tea should be made fresh each day.

Celery seed tea. At least once a day for three days, drink celery seed tea. To prepare the tea, pour one pint of boiling water over a tablespoonful of freshly ground or chopped celery seeds. Let them steep and then cool a bit, strain, and drink. If possible, the tea should be made fresh for each use. Celery seeds increase the elimination of fluid and speed up the clearance of accumulated toxins from the joints, making it beneficial for people with arthritis. For people with excess uric acid, celery seeds can be very helpful as well. These seeds are rich in potassium and sodium, which stimulate the skin, bowels, and kidneys to eliminate waste from the body. They also help to rebalance the body's pH level and may help prevent certain cancers.[4]

Green tea supports the kidneys.

Milk thistle tea supports the kidneys.

Nettles tea is very cleansing for the kidneys. (See Stinging Nettles on page 112 for more information.)

Choose these juices:

Parsley is a good diuretic and often used in kidney cleansing. Mix it with mild-tasting vegetable juices such as celery, carrot, cucumber, and lemon.

Lemon or lime juice. The citric acid in lemon or lime juice may be helpful in reducing calcium levels in the urine, which would reduce the potential of developing calcium kidney stones.[5] Combine 2 tablespoons of freshly squeezed lemon or lime juice and a dash of cayenne pepper in 8 to 10 ounces of purified water. Drink this mixture three times a day for three days. Or you can make lemon-ginger water by adding the juice of one lemon and about 1 tablespoon of fresh ginger juice to a quart of purified water. You should also drink vegetable juices, purified water, and herbal teas as well as eat fresh vegetables and fruits. The goal is to drink at least one gallon of liquid each day.

Cranberry juice. Studies show that cranberry prevents bacteria from adhering to urinary tract walls.[6] Cranberry juice is also very beneficial for cleansing the kidneys. Drink several glasses of unsweetened cranberry juice mixed with water each day. If you can't find fresh cranberries to juice, get premade unsweetened cranberry juice concentrate or unsweetened cranberry juice and add to water according to taste. You may also add fresh lemon juice and a few drops of stevia or a little apple juice to sweeten, if needed.

While you cleanse your kidneys, you may choose (a) to drink only vegetable juice or (b) to drink vegetable juice and eat only raw vegetables and fruits.

As you cleanse and support your kidney and urinary tract, you will expel toxins and waste from your kidneys. The kidney cleanse program can reduce the toxic load on your kidneys, which allows them in turn to do their job of clearing toxins from the bloodstream.

NOTE: If you have a kidney disease, consult your health care professional first. If you suspect kidney stones or have a urinary tract infection, see your doctor immediately.

LIVER CLEANSE

The body stores toxins in the liver, which can't be eliminated well on a standard diet. Many toxic chemicals can pass through the liver, such as residues from pesticides and herbicides. The liver can be damaged by a variety of substances—parasites, chemicals, medications, alcohol, and viruses. And it doesn't take a large dose of toxins or irritating substances to weaken the liver of some individuals who are more susceptible and do not have efficient detoxification systems.

A common medication known to destroy liver cells is acetaminophen (found in Tylenol). Even when a person takes it in recommended amounts, this drug can do great harm to the liver of some people. Fructose is another substance that can scar the liver. Especially avoid high-fructose corn syrup; it is not just a natural sugar made from corn, as commercials would have us believe, but is a damaging substance. Also, agave syrup, which has been very popular as a natural sweetener, is very high in fructose. It is not a good choice in sweeteners as it can damage the liver.

Alcoholics are notorious for having scarred and fatty livers because alcohol is a powerful liver toxin. Over time, heavy drinkers can develop severe scarring of the liver and loss of cells. Chronic heavy drinkers with damaged, poorly functioning livers are also at high risk of liver cancer. This is a result of the chronic scarring, inflammation, and exposure to toxins. But it may not be only heavy drinking that causes problems for some people. Researchers have found even small amounts of alcohol can cause fatty deposits in the livers of susceptible individuals.

Because of our modern diet, many individuals have substantial congestion and even stones in their liver, even though they have not had a history of gallstones. Stones in the liver are an impediment to acquiring and maintaining good health, youthfulness, and vitality. They are, indeed, one of the major reasons people become ill and have difficulty recuperating from illness or recovering from disease.

A congested liver is one reason people have high cholesterol, even though they may eat a very healthful diet and exercise regularly. Your liver creates more cholesterol than a normal diet contains. If you cut your cholesterol intake completely, your body would simply manufacture more. If you have high cholesterol, you may have stones in your liver. As stones grow and congestion increases, the pressure on the liver causes it to make less bile. It could be likened to your garden hose containing pebbles or small stones. Much less water would flow through it, which in turn would decrease the ability of the hose to squirt out water. If you have liver stones, much less bile is "squirted out" and less cholesterol leaves the body, facilitating a rise in cholesterol levels. Taking a medication to bypass the problem and manipulate the numbers is not the answer to healing your body. True preventative medicine means getting to the root cause of the problem and remedying that cause. Performing a liver cleanse will help your liver become more efficient and effective at performing all its functions, including making cholesterol and eliminating cholesterol. Therefore, cleansing your liver is one of the best things you can do to regain balance of your cholesterol

Liver toxicity and congestion are common, but conventional medicine doesn't have a test to determine this. Just relying on a blood test for diagnostic purposes is ineffective. Most people who have liver congestion or stones test perfectly normal for liver enzymes in the blood. Liver enzymes only become elevated when there is advanced liver cell damage, as in hepatitis, cirrhosis, or liver inflammation. That's because liver cells contain large amounts of enzymes, and when they rupture, the enzymes enter the blood and signal liver abnormalities. By then the damage has already occurred. It usually takes many years for this to take place. Therefore cleansing the liver is an excellent preventative measure as well as being healing, restorative, and rejuvenating.

It's difficult to cleanse your liver if you have parasites. You won't be able to release many stones, and you may feel sick. Embark on a parasite-killing program three weeks before attempting a liver cleanse. Also, make sure you complete a colon and kidney cleanse before cleansing the liver. You want your intestinal tract and urinary tract in top working condition so they can efficiently remove waste or toxins.

One of the Best Antiaging Secrets—Avoid Toxins

"The You Docs," Mehmet Oz and Mike Roizen (so named because they are the coauthors of *You, the Owner's Manual*) say, "Give your liver a break: We've long considered toxins—like pollutants in the air and chemical additives in processed foods—major agers, which is what we call things that make your body older faster. When you overload your body with toxins, your liver goes into overdrive trying to filter out the gunk. Over time, excess wear and tear on its filtering system accelerates aging."

So what can you do about the toxins in your life? The You Docs also say, "Treat them the same way you treat toxic people (you know, the ones who drive you to eat that whole cherry cheesecake): Avoid 'em whenever you can. When you can't, help your liver dispose of the vandals."[7]

Symptoms of a Sluggish Liver

Check off the box next to any symptoms you are experiencing. If you have even a few of these symptoms, I recommend a liver cleanse.

- ❏ Abdominal discomfort
- ❏ Aches and pains
- ❏ Allergies
- ❏ Anal itching (may also be a sign of parasites)
- ❏ Bad breath
- ❏ Body odor
- ❏ Brown spots on the face and hands
- ❏ Candidiasis
- ❏ Cellulite
- ❏ Constipation
- ❏ Dark circles under the eyes
- ❏ Digestive problems (belching and/or flatulence)
- ❏ Dizziness
- ❏ Drowsiness after eating
- ❏ Fatigue
- ❏ Frequent urination at night
- ❏ Hemorrhoids
- ❏ Inability to tolerate heat or cold
- ❏ Irritability
- ❏ Loss of memory or inability to concentrate
- ❏ Loss of sexual desire

- ❑ Lower back pain
- ❑ Malaise
- ❑ Menstrual problems
- ❑ Migraine headaches or headaches that involve a feeling of fullness or heaviness in the head
- ❑ Nasal itching (may also be a sign of parasites)
- ❑ Nervousness and anxiety
- ❑ Pain around the right shoulder blade and shoulder (also connected with gallbladder congestion)
- ❑ Premenstrual syndrome
- ❑ Puffy eyes and/or face
- ❑ Red nose
- ❑ Sallow or jaundiced complexion
- ❑ Sinus problems
- ❑ Sleeplessness (insomnia)
- ❑ Small red spots on the skin (either smooth or raised and hard—known as cherry angiomas)
- ❑ Whitish or yellow tongue coating (may also be a sign of candidiasis)

Foods and nutrients that cleanse and support the liver

Optimizing liver function focuses on cleansing, protecting, and nourishing the liver. The following foods and supplements can help you cleanse and support your liver. They are part of a liver cleanse program I describe in my book *Juicing, Fasting, and Detoxing for Life*, which contains recipes including a morning citrus-ginger-olive-oil shake, beet salad, carrot salad, and mineral broth, as well as a menu plan for a seven-day cleansing program.

Liver-friendly vegetables. Juice and eat an abundance of these liver-friendly vegetables during your detoxification program: artichokes, beets, broccoli, brussels sprouts, cabbage, carrots, cauliflower, celery, chives, cucumber, eggplant, garlic, green beans, kale, kohlrabi, lettuce, mustard greens, okra, onion, parsley, parsnips, peas, pumpkin, spinach, squash, and sweet potatoes (yams).

Milk thistle (silymarin). Milk thistle is an herb that protects the liver. Silymarin is the active ingredient in milk thistle, and because of its antioxidant properties, it helps prevent free-radical damage to the liver.

Artichoke powder. A chemical found in artichoke that gives it a bitter taste actually aids your liver in the detoxification process. It helps increase bile production and strengthens the bile duct so that it's better able to contract. The phytochemicals in artichokes also strengthen liver cell walls, protecting them from damage. It also helps break up and mobilize fat stored in the liver, making it useful for lowering cholesterol as well.

Turmeric. The key component in turmeric is curcumin. This golden spice helps cleanse the liver, purify the blood, improve digestion, and promote elimination. It stimulates the gallbladder for bile production and scavenges free radicals.

N-acetyl-L-cysteine (NAC). NAC protects the liver from free-radical damage caused by environmental pollution, radiation, cigarette smoke, and alcohol. Natural health practitioners often prescribe it for patients with mercury or heavy metal toxicity and environmental or dental amalgam mercury-filling toxicity because of its ability to bind to these toxins, allowing your body to excrete them.

L-methionine. L-methionine is an amino acid used by the liver to create glutathione. It can help raise glutathione levels, thus improving the natural detoxification functions of the liver.

Beet leaf and black radish. Beet leaf and black radish assist the liver's detoxification process and improve carbohydrate and fat metabolism. Beet leaf helps normalize the pH of the blood and stimulates bile flow, which can be helpful in lowering cholesterol. Black radish is rich in vitamins and bioflavonoids, which support heavy metal detoxification.

Dandelion. Dandelion has been used for centuries for general detox. Herbalists and naturopathic doctors particularly like dandelion for cleansing the liver. It strengthens the liver by promoting bile secretion and provides a gentle cleansing action in the elimination of metabolic waste. (See the Dandelion section later in this chapter for more information.)

Garlic. Love your liver with garlic. "Use garlic with equal abandon," says Dr. Oz. "In addition to adding oomph to almost any dish, it activates liver enzymes that support your filtration system, and it's good for another vital organ: your heart."[8] Just a small amount of this pungent white bulb has the ability to activate liver enzymes that help your body flush out toxins. Garlic is rich in allicin, the active ingredient, and selenium, two natural compounds that aid in liver cleansing.

Benefits of Cleansing the Liver

- Complexion is clearer and brighter.
- Dark circles disappear from under the eyes.
- Some age spots may disappear.
- Digestion improves.
- Weight loss becomes easier; cellulite goes away.

- Energy increases.
- Sleep improves.
- Aches and pains disappear.
- Headaches often go away.
- Memory improves.
- Mood is better, with a better sense of well-being.
- Allergies go away.
- Facial puffiness disappears.
- Anal and nasal itching stops.
- Body odor goes away.
- Coating on tongue goes away.
- Need to urinate during the night lessens or goes away.
- Sexual desire improves.
- Back pain lessens.
- Nervousness and anxiety go away.
- Facial redness goes away.
- Sinus problems clear up.
- Cellulite improves.
- PMS symptoms lessen.

Liver-cleansing juices

Beet juice. Beets have been used in naturopathic medicine to cleanse and support the liver. Beet juice, made with the root and the leaves, is an integral part of my seven-day liver-cleansing program. It's high in sugar, so always dilute with green veggies like cucumber and dark leafy greens. Also, beet salad is another key part of the program and can be made with the leftover beet pulp and a lemon juice–olive oil dressing. (The recipe is in *Juicing, Fasting, and Detoxing for Life*.)

Carrot juice. Carrots help stimulate and improve overall liver function. They can be juiced as part of the liver-cleansing cocktails. The leftover pulp is made into a cleansing salad with a lemon juice–olive oil dressing. (The recipe is in *Juicing, Fasting, and Detoxing for Life*.)

Dark leafy green juice. One of our most powerful allies in cleansing the liver, leafy greens can be juiced, eaten raw, and lightly cooked. Particularly high in plant chlorophyll, greens literally suck up toxins from the bloodstream. They also halt the progression of hyphae, the long, branching structures of yeast and fungus that cause it to spread systemically throughout the body. And with their distinct ability to neutralize heavy metals, chemicals, and pesticides, greens offer a powerhouse of cleansing for the liver.

Excellent greens to juice include beet tops, arugula, dandelion greens, spinach, mustard greens, kale, chard, collards, kohlrabi leaves, and chicory. Green juice will help increase bile flow, which will help remove waste from the organs and blood.

The olive oil flush for liver and gallbladder cleansing. The olive oil flush is used to purge out stones from the liver and gallbladder. Follow the recipes and program in *Juicing, Fasting, and Detoxing for Life.* For products to cleanse your liver, see Appendix A.

NOTE: If you have a liver disease, consult your doctor first.

Wild Foods and Liver Detoxification (contributed by my dear friend Nina Walsh, ND)

Wild grown greens and herbs offer us some of the most cleansing, medicinal, and nutrient-dense foods we could find. And they are free! Here are some characteristics of wild foods:

- They are organic, clean, resilient, resistant to diseases, and nutrient and antioxidant rich.
- They are grown in rich soils and have greater access to and quality of nutrients
- They come in a variety of species and offer a wide variety of nutrients.
- They have diversity of flavor—bitter, pungent, sour, bland, sweet, and salty.
- They are time-tested—wild plants have been used for thousands of years.
- They have enzyme systems and mechanisms for optimal digestion.
- Our human genome (inherited genetic information) is responsive to wild foods.
- They follow cycles and rhythms of nature, like our bodies.
- They cleanse and nourish our bodies and support optimal health.
- Specific plants cleanse and support specific organs.

Stinging Nettles

The stinging nettle is one of the first plants to come up in early spring. It is used traditionally for body cleansing. People who observe Lent in the Eastern Orthodox tradition abstain from heavy animal foods for about six weeks before Easter and eat spring herbs.

Nettle is a great tonic with unique healing and cleansing qualities. It flushes out toxins and cleanses the entire system. It's best known to detox the kidneys. It helps discharge metabolic wastes, such as uric acid crystals. And it's a good diuretic/aquaretic, meaning it will not waste electrolytes but will get rid of excess water. It gently tones the body, purifying the blood. It also helps cleanse the lymph and rid the body of the residues of months of sedentary winter lifestyle and heavy food. And it replenishes the body with nutrients—it's rich in iron, calcium, beta-carotene, and vitamin C.

In addition to all the cleansing it does, the tea of nettle tops also stimulates the formation of red blood cells. Further, it can lower blood sugar levels and is indicated for type 2 diabetics. This tea can be taken safely by anybody, though it may be particularly supportive for women during puberty, menopause, or pregnancy.

To make the best use of spring nettles, gather young leaves before the plants produce seeds. Use gloves to prevent stinging. You can add them to green smoothies and juice. They will not sting once they are juiced or blended. You can cook them; they are delicious in omelets, sautéed greens, nettle chips, soups, and teas. Also, you can add it to baths, body wash, and hair rinses.

Stinging Nettles Omelet

Start with a bunch of chopped young nettle leaves (use rubber gloves to prepare the nettles). Sauté with shallots or onions in 1 tablespoon of olive oil or coconut oil. Once the nettles are lightly cooked, they'll no longer sting. Add ½ cup sautéed sliced mushrooms and 2 eggs and finish cooking.

Dandelion

Dandelion is the quintessential digestive herb. Its bitter components stimulate production of stomach acid, enhance appetite, support action of the liver in breaking down nutrients, and cleanses the body of toxins. As a liver detox herb, it helps regulate hormones and alleviate hormonal ups and downs, such as those associated with the female menstrual cycle or menopause, and also low vitamin D levels.

One of the best herbs to use for a spring cleanse, dandelion acts as a cleansing agent on both the liver and the kidneys. It helps to purify the blood and flush out uric acid crystals that accumulate from eating a diet too rich in animal proteins and other acid-producing foods; it restores the alkalinity of the blood.

Dandelion enhances bile flow. It also reduces and prevents inflammation in the liver and gallbladder. It contains choline, a substance that helps prevent fat from being deposited in the liver. Dandelion roots are particularly beneficial for the liver, while the leaves have a more pronounced effect on the kidneys as an aquaretic (it does not deplete potassium but actually adds potassium to the body). It is also rich in many other vitamins and minerals, including vitamin C, beta-carotene, calcium, iron, manganese, and phosphorus.

Avoid picking dandelion leaves from lawns where chemical fertilizer was used. It is always best to collect wild foods in clean areas, away from traffic and pesticides.

Every part of this plant can be used as food and medicine. Dandelion can be juiced and added to smoothies. (See Dr. Nina's Sweet Dandelion Smoothie, page 192). For salads, it's best to mix with other milder-tasting spring greens. However, if you don't mind a slightly bitter tang, you can try a dandelion salad with 1 grated carrot and 1–2 cloves garlic. Add a fruity vinaigrette or a sweet and sour dressing made with yogurt, lemon juice, pepper, salt, garlic, and a little raw honey. (Or see Dr. Nina's Russian Cabbage Slaw, page 197.) Dandelion especially complements boiled eggs and cress-type herbs. Like any greens, dandelion leaves and roots can be sautéed or stir-fried. Leaves can also be blended for soups. And you can make "coffee" from roasted roots.

Burdock

One of the best plants for cleansing, burdock is a wonderful digestive herb that supports liver function and detoxification, reduces liver inflammation, heals liver cells in fatty liver disease, and stimulates stomach acid production. It helps lymphatic flow and elimination of wastes from the tissues through the lymphatic system. It is a gentle diuretic and reduces water accumulation in extremities and around joints. It promotes healthy bowel flora and is healing for the intestinal lining. It's also a great source of fiber, protein, vitamins, and minerals.

It can be added to green smoothies and juices. You can use it as you would any root vegetable: sautéed, mixed with greens; added to puréed vegetables; or used in soups. It can be dehydrated as chips or made into a tea. You can also use the leaf and root for infusion for baths

To cook burdock with vegetables: Sauté ½ chopped medium onion in olive oil or coconut oil. Add 1 chopped burdock root, 1 chopped carrot, 1 chopped small beet, 2 chopped Jerusalem artichokes, 1 cup chopped broccoli or another green vegetable (like nettles), 2–3 cloves of chopped garlic, and 2–3 sprigs parsley. Sauté the onion until translucent and then add the rest of the vegetables with chopped garlic. When the vegetables are lightly cooked, add chopped parsley. Salt and pepper to taste. Sprinkle with lemon juice.[9] For more information about Nina Walsh, ND, see Appendix A.

Foods to avoid while cleansing your liver

Omit meat, dairy, sweets, alcohol, eggs, refined foods, sodas, all oils and spreads except olive oil and coconut oil, and all nonorganic foods.

GALLBLADDER CLEANSING

The liver makes bile, and the gallbladder stores and concentrates it until it is required in the small intestines. Bile is made out of cholesterol, water, lecithin, mucin, bile acids, and other organic and inorganic substances. Bile acids are the check-and-balance of this system, designed to keep cholesterol soluble so it doesn't form stones. Our Western diet of high-fat, fiber-depleted, refined foods cause most gallstones or gallbladder congestion, which can trigger abdominal pain, nausea, and vomiting. When bile stagnates in the gallbladder, gallstones can form, leading to possible bacteria growth. This situation often generates gallbladder attacks characterized by severe cramping and pain, particularly if a gallstone blocks the bile duct—the tube connecting the gallbladder to the small intestine. There appears to be an unusually high incidence of gallbladder problems associated with acid reflux (GERD).

You can prevent gallbladder attacks and symptoms of congested gallbladder by periodically cleansing your gallbladder and liver. Also helpful is regularly using curcumin, which stimulates the gallbladder to release its bile. Curcumin has antibacterial and anti-inflammatory properties that help prevent infections and inflammation in this organ.

The cleansing program outlined in my book *Juicing, Fasting, and Detoxing for Life* can help you purge the gallbladder of stones, "sand," or "mud," including the "silent stones" that don't cause symptoms. (The liver and gallbladder will be cleansed at the same time—one program cleanses both.)

Symptoms of Gallbladder Congestion

- Bitter fluid reflux after eating
- Bloating
- Burping or belching
- Constipation—frequent need for laxatives
- Diarrhea (or alternating from soft to watery stools)
- Dizziness
- Feeling of fullness or poor food digestion
- Gas
- Headache over eyes, especially the right eye

- Indigestion after eating (heartburn), especially fatty or greasy foods
- Loss of libido
- Nausea
- Neck and back pain
- Pain between shoulder blades
- Pain or tenderness under the rib cage on the right side
- Stools light or chalky colored

A sound program of periodic detoxification will engage all the major organs in your body's detoxification system—intestines, liver, kidneys, skin, gallbladder, lungs, and lymphatics, to improve your health and prevent disease. You could consider detoxification as being like a thorough spring housecleaning that is taking place on the inside. Just as you need to clean your whole house occasionally and really dig into corners, drawers, and closets where dirt and unwanted items accumulate, so you need to dig deeper when it comes to the organs of elimination and cleanse them thoroughly to eliminate the waste and toxins that have accumulated over time.

Chapter 6

The Living Foods Diet Plan

*If I knew I was going to live this long, I'd
have taken better care of myself.*
—Mickey Mantle

B EFORE YOU GET to the living foods menu plan in the next chapter, I want to guide you in how to make the best food choices possible. This chapter is your shopping guide—your manual of sorts—to lead you through the endless options of unhealthy foodstuffs that line the shelves and freezers of our supermarkets. All animal products are not the same; neither are vegetables and fruit, nor anything else for that matter.

The mission of the living foods revolution is to help you get healthier, lose weight if you need to, detoxify your body, and prevent disease by choosing living foods that are also clean, fresh, whole foods. These are the foods that give your body life. As you learned earlier, you don't have to eat all raw foods to be healthy, but you do need to choose foods that give your body life.

Because the majority of the food in typical grocery stores does not give the body life, smart shopping is the key to healthy eating. And planning ahead is the best way to avoid making poor food choices when there's nothing around to eat and you feel half starved. If you make meal plans and shop ahead of time, you'll have food on hand and an idea for when and how you'll make the food. This will give you a much better chance of succeeding with your living foods lifestyle.

If something unexpected comes your way, have a backup plan for something nutritious you can thaw out, dehydrated foods already made, or something you can quickly put together. To this end the information in this chapter will help you make the wisest choices.

How Many Cheeseburgers Do You Have to Eat to Damage Your Body?

The answer is only one. New research shows that it only takes one "bad" meal such as a burger, fries, and a soda; chicken fried steak with biscuits; or a piece of cake and ice cream to promote a biochemical chain reaction that leads to inflammation of blood vessels and harmful changes to the nervous system, according to James O'Keefe, head of preventive cardiology at the Mid America Heart Institute in Kansas City, Missouri.

As soon as you polish off the last of your high-fat, sugar-rich meal, the sugar causes a large spike in your blood sugar levels called "postprandial hyperglycemia." In the long term this can lead to an increased risk of heart attack, but there are short-term effects as well, which include:

- Inflammation of your tissues (much like when they're infected)
- Constriction of blood vessels
- Generation of free radicals
- Rise in blood pressure

Plus, a spike and drop in insulin may leave you feeling hungry soon after your meal and send you to the fridge not long after you've eaten, which really packs on the pounds.

The desire to eat junk food is a vicious cycle; the more you eat the bad stuff, the more your body craves it. That's because "junk food distorts a person's hormonal profile," according to O'Keefe. It further stimulates your appetite for more unhealthy foods and makes you feel dissatisfied when you eat healthy food.[1]

CHOOSE REAL, WHOLE FOOD

More and more we hear the terms *real foods* or *whole foods*, which is meant to counter substances that are man-made—whipped up in factories and spun out in forms that are anything but real or whole. These foods have become the basis of the American diet, but they should not be called food and should not be part of anyone's diet. They are processed and depleted of natural nutrients and filled with chemicals to promote longer shelf life, ease of transportation, and longer storage. Despite a variety of flavors, textures, and shapes, most of these products are manufactured from the same mono-cultured crops—wheat, corn, soy, and potatoes. They are depleted in nutrients due to growth in high-density environments and depleted soils, while also being saturated with petroleum-based fertilizers. These are among the biggest genetically modified crops (GMO) in America. Due to this stressful growth situation, they are susceptible to pests. Commercial agriculture deals with their susceptibility by spraying them with high amounts of insecticides or by producing GMO frankenplants that have pesticides built in such as Monsanto's Roundup Ready alfalfa. This poses alarming threats to our ecosystem, our long-term food supply, and our health.

Plant nutrient values are further diminished in the course of processing and storage, so the processed foods are fortified with synthetic vitamins and minerals. And flavorings are added to improve the taste because they have very little flavor left. These foods are often addictive and carcinogenic, while being void of nutrients necessary for cellular function. And they deliver empty calories that get stored as fat because the body can't use them for most of its functions.

These products become the basis of disease, obesity, reduced immunity, and reduced fertility, making Americans *the most* overfed and undernourished nation in the world.

Real foods are the foods that are the least processed. They are closest to their natural form and, therefore, retain the most nutrient value and deliver the highest health benefits. They are picked after they've ripened, and they are rich in flavor. They retain natural diversity of taste. They have full nutrient and antioxidant content. And if they are organically grown, seasonal, and local foods, they are the healthiest choices possible.

Fruit, Vegetables, and Legumes

In order to choose the very best fruit, vegetables, and legumes, opt for the freshest food you can find that has been grown organically to avoid toxic pesticides and to get increased nutrition. Buy from local growers whenever possible, because that produce is fresher than anything trucked in from other locations. Many local growers will deliver a box of produce to your door each week. Just check out websites for organic growers in your area. And if you select the produce in season, that's about the freshest food you'll be able to find. And the fresher the produce, the more vitamins and biophotons you'll get.

Vegetables and fruit selected off the shelf at a grocery store usually emit fewer biophotons because of loss during transportation and storage. Chemical, gas, or heat treatment, which is used to ripen or preserve fruits and vegetables, further reduces the amount of biophotons and nutrients available. Irradiation, which is radiation treatment with gamma rays in order to increase the shelf life of food, leads to total destruction of biophotons and many nutrients. (I will discuss irradiation further a little later in this chapter.)

We might be buying attractive fruits and veggies at the market, but their biophoton, enzyme, and vitamin content may be close to zero. For example, avocados may be heat treated in order to speed up ripening, but if the heat is above 110 degrees, it kills enzymes, vitamins, and biophotons—the life force of the cells. Most almonds are required to be pasteurized. But even *raw* almonds may actually have undergone pasteurization, thereby eliminating their biophoton content and reducing their nutrients. The freshest produce can be found at farmers markets, local farms, and your own backyard, along with foraging wild greens. It may be that some day the healthiest food we can find will be unsprayed dandelions in our own backyard.

The quality of protein in vegetables is related to the amount of nitrogen in the soil. Conventional chemical fertilizers add extra nitrogen, which increases the amount of protein but creates a reduction in its quality. Organically managed soils release nitrogen in smaller amounts over a longer time than conventional fertilizers. As a result, the quality of protein from organic crops is better in terms of human nutrition. Indeed, studies show that across the board, organically grown produce is higher in nutrients.[2] (I'll discuss more information on the compelling reasons to purchase organic produce later in this chapter.)

Choose heirloom and wild plants as often as possible. The more of these plants that we eat, the more high-quality nutrition we get. Also, when commercial plants are hybridized, they lose more and more of their inherent biological information contained in the DNA. This is what also makes them more susceptible to the onslaught of diseases, insects, and parasites. Then farmers are told they need to spray their crops with highly toxic chemicals to kill the pests. It's a destructive cycle that affects our health in the end. The more nutrient-rich foods you eat, the more satisfied you'll be and the more cravings will diminish. That will have a positive impact on your health and weight management. Also, this will have positive benefits for farmworkers, the animals, and our earth.

Wild foods. Wild foods like dandelion greens, nettles, burdock, wood sorrel, wild salad greens, and shepherd's purse offer us nutrients found nowhere else. Consider also that if people have adapted to eating wild plants for several hundred thousand years, then problems may arise when we try to eat hybridized and genetically engineered fruits and veggies. Our physiology is just not programmed to handle this.

Vegetables. I encourage you to eat lots of brightly colored vegetables since they are packed with satisfying nutrients. Eat plenty of energy soups, salads, sprouts, vegetable sticks, and steamed vegetables, along with drinking veggie juices and green smoothies and eating raw food dishes. Avoid baked vegetables as much as possible since baking caramelizes the sugars, creating the highest sugar content possible. Limit high-starch vegetables such as potatoes, yams, and winter squash to no more than three times per week if you're trying to lose weight. If you're dining out or it's a special occasion, and you just can't resist a potato, the best choice is red potatoes (less carbs). If you do succumb to a baked potato, which is very high in carbs, eat it with a little fat like butter. This will help to slow down the rate at which sugar enters your blood stream.

Fruit. Four of the best fruits you can choose are lemons, limes (both very alkaline), avocado, and tomato. Avocados are an excellent source of essential fatty acids and glutathione (a powerful antioxidant), along with some protein. They contain more potassium than bananas, making them an excellent choice for heart disorders. Tomatoes are a rich source of vitamin C, beta-carotene, potassium, molybdenum, and one of the best sources of lycopene. The antioxidant function of lycopene includes its ability to help protect cells and other structures in the body from oxygen damage. It has been linked in human research to the protection of DNA (our genetic material) inside of white blood cells. Lycopene also plays a role in the prevention of heart disease. To get the most lycopene, choose organic tomatoes. Lemons and limes are excellent sources of vitamin C and bioflavonoids.

To avoid getting too much sugar, choose the lowest glycemic fruit such as lemons, limes, berries, cantaloupe, cherries, grapefruit, and apples (especially green). Only purchase organic for most of these fruits because they're heavily sprayed. Be aware of eating too much fruit except for lemons and limes. There is an indication that when monkeys only live off of fruit, they start to become hyperactive, like fruitarians. Dr. John Switzer says, "Jean Huntziger, 61, a French raw food adherent for thirty-five years, also came to the conclusion that we need to be careful with (hybrid) sweet fruits and instead, eat more veggies."[3] Cranberries are an excellent low-sugar fruit. Buy them in the fall and freeze some for when they're out of season. They contain iodine, which is good for the thyroid. If you buy store-bought cranberry juice, look for unsweetened cranberry concentrate or pure unsweetened cranberry juice. (Of the bottled juices, cranberry contains the least amount of fungus.) Add lemon, lime, or cranberry juice to flavor water and juices.

Toxic Chemical Approved for Use in California
Despite Health Risks

The chemical methyl iodide has been approved for use on strawberries, nuts, and flowers grown in California despite the fact that the California Office of Environmental Health Hazard Assessment listed the type of toxicity for methyl iodide as "cancer causing" in a document published in 2008. The approval for growers to use this toxin has baffled scientists who know that use of the chemical poses serious risks. It has also spurred communities, advocacy groups, environmental groups, and farmworkers to speak out against the use of this cancer-causing chemical.[4] It is unsettling when our own government allows such harmful practices and citizens have to fight so hard to no avail to keep poisons out of our food. It is even more alarming that the government isn't listening to "we the people."

Legumes (beans, lentils, split peas). Legumes (beans, lentils, dried peas) are packed with nutrition, including protein, calcium, vitamins, and minerals. And they are very cheap. When cooked right, they are delicious. They can also be sprouted. Legumes offer a lot of health benefits. They help prevent food cravings, metabolic syndrome, type 2 diabetes, and obesity. That's because the outer casing of legumes, which is high fiber, slows down the rate at which sugar enters your blood stream. Legumes also protect the body against cancer and heart disease. Further, they provide lots of protein for energy

Why Choose Organic Produce?

The Environmental Protection Agency (EPA) considers 60 percent of herbicides, 90 percent of fungicides, and 30 percent of insecticides to be carcinogenic, and most are damaging to the nervous system as well.[5] Pesticide residues pose long-term health risks, such as cancer, Alzheimer's, Parkinson's, male infertility, miscarriages, and birth defects, along with immediate health risks to farmers and farm workers from acute intoxication like vomiting, diarrhea, blurred vision, tremors, and convulsions.[6]

Many pesticides that are known or suspected to cause brain and nervous system damage, cancer, disruption of the endocrine and immune systems, and a host of other toxic effects are in our food supply. Though the cancer-causing pesticide Alar was banned twenty years ago, we are still no better protected.

In 1996 the federal government finally recognized that vital differences did exist for children and passed the Food Quality Protection Act, which required the EPA to reassess the nearly five hundred pesticide chemicals that come in contact with food in order to test their safety for children. But five years later, the EPA had reviewed only about one hundred chemicals. They decided that more than half of them could be left unchanged.[7] The only way to protect yourself and your children or grandchildren is to buy organic produce, except for those items that are rated very low (the Clean Fifteen) on the pesticide-sprayed list of the safest foods rated by the Environmental Working Group.

There is a far greater incidence of cancer, particularly lymphoma, leukemia, and cancer of the brain, skin, stomach, and prostate among farmers, their families, and farmworkers when compared with cancer rates among the general public.[8] This data alone should be alarming enough to ban all pesticides in America. But there are huge profits at stake for big corporations that lobby hard in Washington, pay for studies to show that their pesticides aren't that harmful, and "educate" farmers on the merits of pesticides, making them believe that we would not have enough food to feed people if it weren't for pesticides.

This is far from true. Our local co-op (PCC) published an excellent article in their *Sound Consumer* paper in September 2010 titled "Organic Can Feed the World." Author Maria Rodale states, "Biotech and chemical companies have spent billions of dollars trying to make us think that synthetic fertilizers, pesticides, and genetically modified organisms (GMO) are necessary to feed a growing population. But science indicates otherwise. There's clear and conclusive scientific data showing organic agriculture is key not only to solving global hunger but also to... promoting public health, revitalizing farming communities, and restoring the environment."[9]

Research by the Rodale Institute called the Farm System Trail (FTS), which began in 1981, shows that once soil is restored organically from depletion due to years of mismanagement, organic crops yield comparable to yields using chemicals. The study also found that organic farm yields are higher during times of drought and floods due to stronger root systems and better moisture retention. The FTS data also showed that organic production requires 30 percent less energy than chemical production for growing corn and soybeans. They also found that organic production stores a great deal of carbon and concluded that if we returned globally to organic farming, we could reduce our CO_2 pollution significantly. These findings are supported by the $12 million study by the International

Assessment of Agricultural Knowledge, Science, and Technology for Development.[10]

When you purchase produce from certified organic farmers or from local farmers who sell unsprayed produce but are working without certification, you won't get synthetic fertilizers, sewage sludge, genetically modified organisms, or ionizing radiation. Buying your vegetables from a local source is also the best way to insure freshness. Keep in mind that the fresher the vegetables and fruit, the more biophotons you'll be receiving. Many local farmers will deliver a box of organic produce each week for a very reasonable price. We have fresh organic veggies delivered to our door, and it's always a nice surprise to see what we'll get that week. The vegetables we get differ from week to week. If you sign up for such a program, there may be items in the box you've never eaten before, which is great! You'll get to try something new. And that's the best way to get maximum nutrition—by varying your foods and not eating the same things all the time.

Is Organic Food More Nutritious?

It's often questioned if organic produce is more nutritious than conventionally grown fruits and vegetables. Studies have shown that it is. According to results from a $25 million study into organic food, the largest of its kind to date, organic produce completely surpasses conventional produce in nutritional content. A four-year, European Union–funded study in 2007 found that organic fruits and vegetables contain up to 40 percent more antioxidants. They have higher levels of beneficial minerals like iron and zinc. Milk from organic herds contained up to 90 percent more antioxidants. The researchers obtained their results after growing fruits and vegetable, and raising cattle on adjacent organic and nonorganic sites attached to Newcastle University. According to Professor Carlo Leifert, coordinator of the project, eating organic foods can significantly help to increase the nutrient intake of people who don't eat the recommended number of servings of fruits and vegetables a day.[11]

Additionally, a 2001 study completed as part of a doctoral dissertation at Johns Hopkins University looked at forty-one different studies involving field trials, greenhouse pot experiments, market basket surveys, and surveys of farmers. The most studied nutrients across those surveys included calcium, copper, iron, magnesium, manganese, phosphorus, potassium, sodium, zinc, beta-carotene, and vitamin C. Many studies also looked at nitrates. According to the study, there was significantly more vitamin C (27 percent), iron (21 percent), magnesium (29 percent) and phosphorus (13 percent) in the organic produce than in the conventionally grown vegetables. There were also 15 percent fewer nitrates in the organic vegetables. The vegetables that had the largest increases in nutrients between organic and conventional production were lettuce, spinach, carrots, potatoes, and cabbage.[12] Couple that with fewer chemical residues, and you can see that buying organically grown food is well worth the effort and the additional cost. Plus, you're investing in sustainability of farming and the health of the entire human community as well as our earth.

Buying Organic: How to Choose the Best

When choosing organically grown foods, look for labels that are marked *certified organic*. This means the produce has been cultivated according to strict uniform standards that are verified by independent state or private organizations. Certification includes inspection of farms and processing facilities, detailed record keeping, and pesticide testing of soil and water to ensure that growers and handlers are meeting government standards. But there are a couple of categories where there's evidence that standards may be getting lax with dairy products and the labeling of some packaged foods.

Support your local farms and farmers who sell their produce at farmers markets, local markets, and home deliveries. Many of the smaller farms can't promote their wares as "organic," but if you talk with them, you'll learn that they don't use pesticides or chemical fertilizers; they just can't afford to get certified.

You may occasionally see a label that says *transitional organic*. This means that the produce was grown on a farm that recently converted or is in the process of converting from chemical sprays and fertilizer to organic farming. It's always a good idea to support these farmers.

One Reason to Always Purchase Organic

There is indication that organophosphates may be a causal factor in bovine spongiform encephalopathy (BSE, known as "mad cow disease") and Creutzfeldt-Jakob Disease (CJD, a rare and usually fatal brain disease), and they are a contributing factor in Alzheimer's disease. If this truth really gets communicated to the masses, millions of people may stop buying conventional produce altogether.

The switch to organophosphates happened after the toxic effects of organochlorine pesticides were discovered. Organophosphates now represent the majority of insecticides and herbicides in use—affecting more than 90 percent of US produce and representing huge profits for the chemical giants.[13]

Most nonorganic produce today has measurable residues of organophosphate pesticides. There is evidence that these pesticides may be contributing to major diseases such as Alzheimer's and Parkinson's. Serious health concerns regarding this class of pesticides also place the genetic engineering of crops into question because the use of these pesticides is necessary for their survival.

COMPLETELY AVOID IRRADIATED FOODS

Nonorganic vegetables, meats, and other products have been irradiated for years. Irradiation kills insects and other bugs that may have crawled into foods before being shipped to the grocery store. From apples to zucchini, produce is routinely irradiated. It may seem that food irradiation to kill bacteria and bugs on nonorganic vegetables and meat should be beneficial. Most people would think that spinach irradiated to kill salmonella is happy spinach, right? Not necessarily.

Here's what's really going on. In order to kill all these insects, bacteria, fungus, and mold, and to give food a longer shelf life, food is exposed to radiation in very high levels. In the United States this practice began in the 1960s with the irradiation of wheat and white potatoes. Since then the FDA has approved a steady stream of foods for irradiation: in the 1980s, spices and seasonings, pork, fresh fruit, and dried and dehydrated substances were approved; in 1990, poultry; and in 1997, red meat was approved.[14]

Irradiation has been shown to produce chromosome damage. Studies performed with children in Hyderabad, India, by the National Institute of Nutrition at the Council of Medical Research showed chromosome damage after being fed freshly irradiated wheat for six weeks. Other children who were fed a similar diet that was not irradiated did not show chromosome damage. The condition gradually reversed when the children were taken off the irradiated diet.[15]

Irradiation also causes nutrient destruction. It destroys essential vitamins, including vitamin A; thiamine; vitamins B_2, B_3, B_6, and B_{12}; folic acid; and vitamins C, E, and K. Amino acid and essential fatty acid content may also be harmed. A 20 to 80 percent loss of these nutrients is common. Also, irradiation kills friendly bacteria and enzymes, rendering the food "dead" and useless to the body—the opposite of a living foods diet. And it can generate harmful by-products such as free radicals, which are toxins that can damage cells, and harmful chemicals known as *radiolytic products*, including formaldehyde and benzene.[16]

The answer to food-borne illnesses is not irradiation; the answer is stopping the overuse of pesticides, adopting sustainable organic farming practices, transforming overcrowded factory-farm animal lots to humane sanitary farms, and ensuring more sanitary conditions in food-processing plants.

The only good thing is that in the United States, food growers and manufacturers must put the irradiation symbol on the label that the food is irradiated, so avoidance of irradiated foods is possible if one shops carefully. Since 1986, all irradiated products must carry the international symbol called a *radura*, which is a flower within a circle. But it is similar to the symbol for the Environmental Protection Agency. Whenever you see this radura symbol (stylized flower), complain to your supermarket manager. However, if you eat out, you will not know when you're eating irradiated food, since restaurants are not obliged to reveal that information to their customers. You can ask the server or manager, but they may not know. Some restaurants refuse to serve irradiated food, while others serve it regularly.

Say No to GMO

What do tortilla chips, soymilk, and canola oil have in common? They're all made from the top GMO crops in North America.

Of the more than fifty genetically modified (GM) plant varieties that have been examined and approved for human consumption, the majority of them are modified for herbicide tolerance and pest tolerance[17]—for example, tomatoes and cantaloupes have modified ripening characteristics; soybeans and sugar beets are resistant to herbicides; and corn and cotton plants have increased resistance to insect pests.

There are other foods to watch for and buy only organic. Rice is modified to boost its vitamin A levels. Sugar cane is genetically modified to resist pesticides. A large percentage of sweeteners used in processed food actually come from corn, not sugar cane or beets, and corn is one of the biggest GM crops in America. Beets were recently approved as a GM crop. GM papayas now make up about three quarters of the total Hawaiian papaya crop. Meat and dairy products often come from animals that have been fed or injected with GM products, which is why it's very important to purchase only pasture-fed, organically raised animal products. Genetically modified peas have created immune responses in mice, suggesting that they could also create serious allergic reactions in people. Peas had a gene inserted from kidney beans, which creates a protein that acts as a pesticide.[18] Many vegetable oils and margarines used in restaurants and in processed foods and salad dressings are made from soy, corn, canola, or cottonseed. Unless these oils specifically say "Non-GMO" or "organic," they are probably genetically modified.

When trying to avoid the top GM crops, you'll need to watch out for maltodextrin, soy lecithin, soy oil, textured vegetable protein (soy), canola oil, corn products, and high-fructose corn syrup. Other GM crops to avoid include some varieties of zucchini, crookneck squash, papayas from Hawaii, aspartame (NutraSweet), milk containing rbGH, and rennet (containing genetically modified enzymes) used to make hard cheeses. Many of these products you would not want anyway, but when it comes to these foods, unless you buy organically grown, it's quite probable you'll be eating genetically modified food. And that should cause you great concern.

Even vitamin supplements may be genetically modified or contain GM material. For example, vitamin C is often made from corn (look for "non-corn source" on the label), and vitamin E is usually made from soy. Vitamins A, B_2, B_6, B_{12}, D, and K may have fillers derived from GM corn sources, such as starch, glucose, and maltodextrin.[19] This is precisely the reason for purchasing only high-quality vitamins from reliable sources that use organic materials.

We must become informed consumers and careful shoppers. We can look at the labels of packaged products to see if they contain corn flour or cornmeal, soy flour, cornstarch, textured vegetable protein (TVP), corn syrup, or modified food starch. Check labels of soy sauce, tofu, soy beverages, soy protein isolate, soymilk, soy ice cream, soy cheese, margarine, and soy lecithin, among dozens of other products. If it doesn't say organic or non-GMO, don't buy it; the chances are strong that they are GMO. To shop smart, see the Non-GMO Shopping Guide, created by the Institute for Responsible Technology, at www.nongmoshoppingguide .com.

When we refuse to buy GMO products, we will also help to reduce pollution. A variety of noxious gases are polluting our world, and nitrous oxide (N_2O) makes up 10 percent of them. This gas is three hundred times more destructive than CO_2 and has the ability to remain in the atmosphere almost permanently. Two-thirds of this gas emission comes from nitrate fertilizers used on GM industrial farms. The largest GMO crops that utilize them are those grown with billions of tons of pesticides for factory farms and feedlots.[20]

Currently the FDA does not require that foods be labeled GMO. But without protective labeling, we will not know when we are buying them because GM foods look just like non-GM foods. And unsuspecting consumers are eating products that have the potential to damage their health. The only way to avoid GM foods is by becoming aware of which foods are genetically engineered and what products are made from them, and purchase only organic foods and products made from those foods. Some estimates reveal that as many as thirty thousand different products on grocery store shelves are genetically modified, which is largely because many processed foods contain some form of soy.

WISE UP ABOUT RED MEAT

Not all red meat is created equal. In addition to being higher in omega-3 fats and CLA, meat from grass-fed animals is also higher in vitamin E. In fact, studies show the meat from pastured cattle is four times higher in vitamin E than meat from feedlot cattle and, interestingly, almost twice as high as the meat from feedlot cattle given vitamin E supplements. That's beneficial, in that vitamin E is linked with a lower risk of heart disease and cancer.[21]

Grass-fed beef is also lower in total fat and particularly the saturated fats linked to heart disease. It's also higher in beta-carotene, the B vitamins thiamine and riboflavin, and the minerals calcium, magnesium, and potassium.

A team of scientists from the USDA compared grass-fed lambs with lambs fed grain in a feedlot. They found that lambs grazing on pasture had 14 percent less fat and about 8 percent more protein compared to grain-fed lamb. And check this out! Meat from sheep raised on pasture has shown twice as much lutein (carotene) as meat from grain-fed sheep. Lutein reduces the risk of cataracts and macular degeneration (a leading cause of blindness) and may also help prevent breast and colon cancer.[22]

PASTURED POULTRY VERSUS FREE-RANGE OR COMMERCIAL FOWL

Pasture-raised poultry are far healthier than commercial-raised fowl. Pastured poultry are chickens, turkey, ducks, and geese that are raised in bottomless cages or pens outside or on grass where they can peck and scratch at the ground and hunt for bugs and seeds along with their grain. They breathe fresh air and roam in the sun. Their manure is spread over wide areas of pasture as they are moved, which is good for the soil as well as the birds.

Sometimes they are mistakenly called free-range chickens, but free-range birds are still kept in confinement; they are just allowed to roam inside their buildings, which are often very crowded so "roaming" is not really possible.

Commercially raised factory farm birds fare the worst. They are housed in small cages where they can't even turn around with their feet standing in their own manure from birth to death. They do not get the benefits of fresh air and sunshine or the grass, seeds, and bugs of the pasture they are meant to eat. They are stressed, drugged, and sick most of their lives.

When you choose pasture-raised chicken, you avoid the following:

- *Hormones, antibiotics, and drugs.* There is growing concern that hormone and drug residues in muscle meats, eggs, and milk might be harmful to human health and the environment. There may be immunological effects and cancer risks for consumers.[23]
- *Arsenic.* Commercial poultry are often fed trace amounts of arsenic in their feed to stimulate their appetites so they'll fatten quickly for market. Traces of arsenic can be found in the meat we buy.[24]

Eggs From Pastured Hens

Eggs contain all eight essential amino acids and are a rich source of essential fatty acids, especially when raised on pasture. They also contain considerably more lecithin (a fat emulsifier) than cholesterol. Additionally, eggs from hens bred outdoors have four to six times more vitamin D than eggs from hens bred in confinement.[25] Pastured hens are exposed to direct sunlight, which is converted to vitamin D and passed on to the eggs. And the eggs are rich in sulfur and glutathione as well.

Look for eggs from chickens that are raised cage-free on pasture, without hormones, and fed an organic diet that includes green grass. When chickens are housed indoors and deprived of greens, their eggs become low in good fats.

For organic pastured eggs, look to co-ops and natural food markets; also seek out local producers, farmers, and homesteaders who pasture their poultry in movable pens or let them roam free.

Lab Tests on Eggs From Pastured Chickens

Mother Earth News collected samples from fourteen pastured chicken flocks across the country and had them tested at an accredited laboratory. The results were compared to official USDA data for commercial eggs. Results showed the pastured eggs contained an astounding:

- One-third less cholesterol than commercial eggs
- One-fourth less saturated fat
- Two-thirds more vitamin A
- Two times more omega-3 fatty acids
- Seven times more beta-carotene[26]

WILD FISH VERSUS FARM RAISED

To select the best fish, buy only wild-caught—meaning caught with a boat and hook or net. The other option is ranched or farm-raised fish, which you should avoid. Farm-raised fish are housed within small pens that are set up in the ocean or in small ponds. The fish are often kept in overcrowded conditions that increase their risk of infection and disease. Instead of being allowed to find their own natural food sources (other fish and krill), they're fed dried food pellets made up of fish oil and fish meal containing concentrations of toxins, chicken feces, corn meal, soy, genetically modified canola oil, and other fish. The dried food pellets are often contaminated with such cancer-causing agents as PCBs, dioxins, and even flame-retardants. This creates a very unnatural environment, which yields unhealthy fish. In fact, because their flesh looks anemic, these fish are given artificial colorings in their food to get the same coloration back that wild salmon have naturally.

Because farm-raised fish are susceptible to disease due to their overcrowded living conditions and very poor diet, they're often given antibiotics, which become part of their flesh. Some sources say that salmon are given more antibiotics than farm animals. In contrast, wild salmon are relatively free of these substances and disease.

Farm-raised fish do not have the essential fatty acids that wild-caught fish offer and that are so important for our health. When it comes to animal fat, wild-caught fish are a good source of the healthy omega-3 fatty acids, especially coldwater fish such as salmon, mackerel, and trout. Also, the smaller the fish, the less mercury and other heavy metals that will be stored in the flesh and fat.

VEGETABLE JUICE, TEA, AND OTHER BEVERAGES

Freshly made raw, vegetable juices are alkaline producing. Avoid processed fruit juices; they become more acid producing when processed and especially when sweetened. Fresh vegetable juices are an integral part of your living foods lifestyle regimen because they promote health in a variety of ways. The concentration of vitamins, minerals, phytonutrients, biophotons, and enzymes that juicing provides gives the body extra stamina and boosts the immune system.

As I explained in chapter 2, freshly made vegetable juice, and especially green juice, is the core of *The Juice Lady's Living Foods Revolution*. My recommendation is that you drink two glasses of veggie juice each day. It's best to drink one glass of veggie juice in the morning and one in the afternoon or before dinner. The morning juice helps energize your body and gives you super nutrients to last all morning; the afternoon juice is a pick-me-up for the afternoon slump many people experience, and/or the evening juice (before dinner cocktail) helps curb your appetite and gives you energy to make a healthy dinner. If this schedule isn't possible, then drink the juices whenever you can.

You can make them the night before and take juice to work in a stainless steel water bottle or thermos. You can store juice in a covered container in the refrigerator up to twenty-four hours. It won't lose all its nutrients as some say, although the longer juice sits, the more nutrients it loses. I recovered from chronic fatigue syndrome by juicing once a day and making enough juice to last for twenty-four hours until I had the strength to juice the next afternoon. I know I didn't lose a large amount of the nutrients.

Green tea is a great addition to your healthy lifestyle. Rich in antioxidants and the phytonutrients catechins and other polyphenols that protect against inflammation, cancer, and other ailments, green tea is also thermogenic. Thermogenesis is the production of heat, meaning that it revs up your metabolism. Most of the thermogenic action in green tea is due to epigallocatechin gallate (EGCG), which is a potent polyphenol. For these reasons it's a great idea to make green tea part of your daily meal plan. Strive for at least one cup of organic green tea per day. A cup of green tea has about one-third of the caffeine found in a cup of coffee. Avoid green tea if you are sensitive to caffeine, have low adrenal function, or are hypoglycemic.

White tea has less caffeine than green tea and may be better tolerated. Herbal teas are also a great choice and are fine for those with low adrenal function and who are hypoglycemic. When choosing green, white, and herbal tea, look for organically grown. And unbleached tea bags are a better choice over bleached.

For sparkling water, choose mineral water that is naturally carbonated such as S. Pellegrino and Apollinaris over commercially gassed varieties, If you suffer from IBS, Crohn's disease, celiac, or diverticulitis, it is advisable to completely eliminate carbonated drinks along with all gluten from your diet in order to allow the GI lining of your intestinal tract to heal.

Be sure to drink plenty of water. It's recommended that you drink at least eight 8-ounce glasses of purified water per day for weight loss and to maintain good health. A good water purifier is a great investment. Be aware of plastic toxins that are leached into the water from plastic bottles. Take water with you in stainless steel water bottles.

Completely avoid soft drinks; they are like drinking liquid candy with chemicals so caustic they can rust nails. They're loaded with sugar or artificial sweeteners, which are even worse. Studies have connected them with weight gain and numerous health problems. They're also very acidic. Also, watch out for sweetened teas, energy drinks, sports drinks, and vitamin-infused water. And always avoid diet sodas due to their detrimental health effects and the fact that studies show artificial sweeteners actually cause people to gain weight.[27]

Fats and Oils

For decades we've have had a love-hate relationship with this food that makes so many dishes taste great. Fat gives us that feeling of satisfaction we all long for—satiety, which is the sense that we've had enough to eat. But that's not all. Fats play an important role in our body's health. Some fats can even help us lose weight. Unfortunately, we consume too few of the healthy fats and too many of the unhealthy man-made versions.

It's difficult to eat enough food on a low-fat diet to get the energy we need. Fat provides that energy. Essential fats like fish oils are brain food—a deficiency can lead to numerous health and psychiatric/social problems. We need fats to absorb fat-soluble vitamins such as A, D, E, and K. But which fats are the best choices? Which fats can be harmful to our bodies? And which ones, because of their chemical processing, have the most negative impact on our health and the environment?

Since the 1950s we've been told to use vegetable oil for heart health. It looks clear and pure in a bottle on your shelf. No worries, right? Oh, so wrong. We've been led astray. Polyunsaturated oils (corn, safflower, sunflower, soy, cottonseed) are especially susceptible to oxidation because they have more than one double bond, which can be broken rather easily when exposed to heat, sunlight, and oxygen. This is why they have the greatest tendency to oxidize. This triggers inflammation, a leading cause of heart disease, and can damage blood vessels Oxidation can happen even in the processing of these oils, and it is accelerated with heat, which they undergo in processing unless they are cold processed. The oils are then deodorized, which means that we can't smell when they are rancid. Rancid oil generates free radicals, which are produced in the processing and are one of the primary causes of oxidized cholesterol. It is oxidized cholesterol that is implicated in heart disease, not general LDL. This is the reason unsaturated fats are so dangerous. There should be a warning on every label so consumers can make an educated purchase, but then that would curtail profits.

Oxidized oils also damage cells, causing inflammation. Inflammation produces insulin resistance, and insulin resistance produces weight gain. Weight gain generates inflammatory cytokines, leading to more insulin resistance and more weight gain. It becomes a frustrating cycle of gaining more and more weight.

When people eat foods prepared with processed vegetable oils—margarine, french fries, fried food, nonfat dried milk, powdered or liquid coffee creamer, many salad dressings, crackers, cookies, chips, and a plethora of processed and convenience foods—they eat a high quantity of oxidized (rancid) oil. This sets the body up for heart disease and numerous other health problems.

To help you choose the very best oils and fats, the following is your shopping guide for the healthiest fats and oils, along with the ones to avoid. I've also included the smoke point of the oils recommended, which is the point at which fat breaks down, starts to smoke, and gives off an odor, signaling the oxidation of these oils.

Coconut oil. Choose only organic virgin coconut oil, which means it has been made by a traditional method that does not involve high heat or harmful chemicals. It won't oxidize (turn rancid) as easily because it doesn't have the double bonds that make polyunsaturated oils most vulnerable to oxidation. It has a longer shelf life (about two years) than most oils and does not need to be refrigerated. It has been a staple cooking oil for thousands of years in tropical climates. It is white when solid, creamy colored when liquid.

Many commercial-grade coconut oils are made from copra, which means the dried kernel (meat) of the coconut. If standard copra is used as a starting material, the unrefined coconut oil extracted from copra is not suitable for human consumption and must be refined. This is because most copra is dried under the sun in the open air in very unsanitary conditions where it's exposed to insects and molds. Though producers may start with organic coconuts and even label their coconut oil organic, the end product of some brands is refined, bleached, and deodorized oil. High heat and chemical solvents are usually used in this process. If you select virgin coconut oil made by hand the old-fashioned way, you will immediately notice the difference in taste, smell, and texture from oil made with standard copra. The traditionally made oil, which is known as virgin coconut oil, is far superior in every way. You will pay more for this oil, but it's well worth it.

Research has shown that coconut oil can help you lose weight—the body likes to burn its medium-chain fatty acids rather than store them as it does long-chain fatty acids that dominate many other oils.[28] It has a "thermogenic effect," meaning it raises body temperature, thus boosting energy and metabolic rate and promoting weight loss. It has also been shown in a university study to kill yeasts, even Candida albicans.[29]

Coconut oil is great for medium-heat cooking (smoke point of 350 degrees). It has no cholesterol, which some have claimed. And it tastes great on popcorn.

Olive oil is an outstanding monounsaturated fat. A tablespoon of extra-virgin olive oil contains 11 grams of monounsaturated fat, 2 grams of saturated fat and 1 gram of polyunsaturated fat. An ancient oil dating back to biblical times, it was used for cooking and healing. It is more shelf stable than polyunsaturated oils. The most flavorful, healthful, and eco-friendly varieties are extra-virgin, organic oils that are cold-pressed or expeller-pressed. These are produced without chemical solvents like hexane and high heat. High-quality olive oil stands out also as an antioxidant that is a free-radical fighter.

Olive oil is great for salad dressings, cold foods, and low-heat cooking such as light sautéing. Extra-virgin olive oil has a smoke point of 305–320 degrees. Other monounsaturated oils such as avocado and almond oil are better suited for higher-heat cooking.

Completely avoid the less expensive, chemically derived version called olive pomace oil—the last dregs of the olive oil pressing process, extracted by petroleum solvents such as hexane.

Almond oil is monounsaturated oil that is extracted from the almond and has a distinctively nutty flavor. It is typically used as an ingredient in salad dressings, sauces, mayonnaise, and desserts. Unlike almond extract, almond oil is not concentrated enough to provide a strong almond taste.

It is suited for high-heat cooking and baking with a smoke point of 420 degrees. Many toxic pesticides and herbicides are used on almond trees; therefore, choose only organic cold-pressed or expeller-pressed almond oil.

Avocado oil is extracted from the avocado by pressing the flesh, not the seed. It is often compared to olive oil because the oils are similar in composition, but avocado oil has a much higher smoke point of 520 degrees and is good for high-heat cooking and baking. High-quality avocado oil has a distinct green color due to its chlorophyll content. It also has a characteristic avocado flavor, depending on how the oil has been processed and handled and the quality of the avocados used. Avocado oil is fairly shelf stable and does not oxidize easily. Choose cold-pressed or expeller-pressed avocado oil. Avoid chemically processed oil altogether.

Rice bran oil is extracted from the germ and inner husk of rice. It is dominantly monounsaturated. A tablespoon contains 7 grams of monounsaturated fat, 3 grams of saturated fat, and 5 grams of polyunsaturated fat. It contains healthful phytochemicals such as beta-sitosterol, which can reduce the absorption of cholesterol, and alpha-linoleic acid, which can increase essential fatty acid concentration.

Rice bran oil has a mild taste and is popular in Asian cuisine because of its suitability for high-temperature cooking such as stir-frying, with a smoke point of 490 degrees. It is said to be the secret of good tempura. Rice bran oil also contains components of vitamin E that may benefit health and prevent rancidity. Look for organic, cold-pressed or expeller-pressed oil.

Peanut oil (unrefined) has a smoke point of 320 degrees, which makes it good for only low-heat cooking. Refined peanut oil has a much higher smoke point but is not recommended because of being refined. Peanut oil contains 48 percent monounsaturated fat, 18 percent saturated fat, and 34 percent polyunsaturated fat. Like olive oil, peanut oil is relatively stable and, therefore, appropriate for stir-fry. But the high percentage of omega-6 fatty acids it contains presents a potential problem since the American diet contains far too much omega-6 already and not enough omega-3 fats. Limit your use of peanut oil, and choose only organic, cold-pressed, or expellier-pressed, or better yet, avoid it altogether since peanuts are grown underground and known to absorb toxins from the soil.

Sesame oil contains 42 percent monounsaturated fat, 15 percent saturated fat, and 43 percent polyunsaturated fat. It has been used for thousands of years in Asian culture. Sesame oil is similar in composition to peanut oil. The high percentage of omega-6 fats indicates that it should be used only occasionally in small quantities. Hexane is typically used to extract oil from the seeds, so choose only cold-pressed or expeller-pressed oil, and always refrigerate it. Organic is better, but pesticide residues are minor in nonorganic sesame seeds and oils.

Macadamia nut oil is expressed from the meat of the macadamia. Native to Australia, the oil contains approximately 60 percent monounsaturated fat, about 20 percent saturated fat, and 20 percent polyunsaturated fat. Some varieties contain roughly equal omega-6s and omega-3s. It is very shelf stable due to its low polyunsaturated fat content. It has a smoke point of 410 degrees, making it suitable for higher-heat cooking. Few pesticides are used on these nuts, so organic oil is not necessary. But choose only cold-pressed or expeller-pressed oil because the highest concentration of hexane residue was found in macadamia nut oil in a study that tested 41 samples of vegetable, fruit, and nut oils.[30]

Butter. Purchase organic butter from grass-fed cows. It has more cancer-fighting conjugated linoleic acid (CLA), vitamin E, beta-carotene, and omega-3 fatty acids than butter from cows raised on factory farms or that have limited access to pasture. A 2006 study showed that the cows who ate the most fresh grass had the softer butter. Cows that eat only grass have the softest butterfat of all—a sign you're getting the best butter.[31]

Butter is dominated by short- and medium-chain fatty acids. It's a healthier choice than margarine or most other vegetable spreads, with the exception of coconut oil and olive oil spreads. Butter is a rich source of vitamins A, E, K, and D. It also has appreciable amounts of butyric acid, which is used by the colon as an energy source, and lauric acid, a medium-chain fatty acid that is a potent antimicrobial and antifungal substance. Butter from grass-fed cows also contains CLA, which gives excellent protection against cancer and helps us lose weight. Because living grass is richer in vitamins E, A, and beta-carotene than stored hay or standard diets for dairy cows, butter from dairy cows grazing on fresh pasture is also richer in these important nutrients. The naturally golden color of grass-fed butter is a good indication of its superior nutritional value.[32]

Butter is suited for medium-heat cooking with a smoke point of 350 degrees. Ghee, which is clarified butter, has a smoke point between 375 and 485 degrees and is good for medium- to high-heat cooking.

Avoid These Foods Completely

Polyunsaturated oils. In their natural state, as found in nuts, vegetables, and seeds, polyunsaturated fats are healthy. But when they are processed into oil, they oxidize easily and do more harm than good. In the past half century, the ratio of omega-6 fats, from polyunsaturated oils (corn, safflower, sunflower, cottonseed, and soybean oils), to omega-3 fats has changed in the Western diet from 2:1 to 14 to 25:1, which promotes inflammation that leads to weight gain, depression, and immune system dysfunction. Our diets now include too few omega-3s, which are found primarily in wild-caught fish, fish oil, seafood, grass-fed meat and dairy, walnuts, flax, hemp, and chia seeds, and in smaller amounts in vegetables, whole grains, and beans.

Canola oil is a monounsaturated fat, as is olive oil, which means it contains only one double bond, so technically it could be used for salad dressings, cold food preparation, and low-temperature cooking. But there's a major reason not to use it: most canola oil comes from GM crops. Also, researchers at the University of Florida at Gainesville found trans fat levels as high as 4.6 percent in processed canola oil.[33]

Trans fats are created in the process of hydrogenating oils and should be avoided completely. The consumption of trans fats increases the risk of coronary heart disease. Commercially baked goods such as crackers, cookies, cakes, muffins, and many fried foods, such as doughnuts and french fries, may contain trans fats. Mainstream shortenings and some margarine can be high in trans fat.

Margarine and butter replacement spreads. Margarine is made from different types of oils mixed with emulsifiers, vitamins, coloring, flavoring, and other ingredients. The oils often are hydrogenated—a process used to solidify them, making the margarine solid and spreadable. The *New York Times* says, "A new report by Harvard researchers says a fat [trans fat] in margarine and other processed foods could be responsible for 30,000 of the nation's annual deaths from heart disease."[34] When it comes to natural spreads that are substitutes for butter, read labels; know what oils are used. An olive oil or coconut oil spread would be fine, but anything made with polyunsaturated oils or canola oil (unless it specifically says non-GMO/no trans fats) should be avoided.

Salt. Choose only Celtic sea salt, Himalayan pink, or gray salt. Whole sea salt has a mineral profile that is similar to our blood. Regular table salt is highly refined sodium chloride that usually contains additives to make it pour easily. When salt is processed, minerals are removed. Then, anti-caking chemicals such as potassium oxide or aluminum calcium silicate, iodine, and dextrose (sugar) are added to make table salt. Eat salt sparingly, even Celtic, pink, or gray salt as it causes the body to retain water.

Sugar—all types. Most of the sugar we eat is disguised in sodas and other drinks, desserts, boxed cereals, energy bars, packaged foods, snacks, and yogurt. Much of it is high-fructose corn syrup, which is used to sweeten everything from crackers, tomato sauces, ketchup, sodas, processed meats, and even some health food products. It's used primarily because it's cheap. But many health professionals attribute it to the increase in obesity, metabolic syndrome, diabetes, certain cancers, and heart disease. The more you avoid sugar, the less you will crave it. And you'll lose weight!

Check out the website www.sugarshock.com. You'll learn about journalist Connie Bennett's journey to a changed life by avoiding sugar. She suffered from dozens of debilitating symptoms for years. Finally a doctor connected her condition to overeating processed carbohydrates and sweets, which included her favorites—red licorice, chocolate, and hard candy.

All of these sugar sources need to be avoided: high-fructose corn syrup; sucrose (white sugar—another big GMO product), brown sugar (white sugar with molasses added), dextrose (produced synthetically from starch), honey, dextrin (a complex sugar molecule, left over from enzyme action on starch), sugar alcohols such as sorbitol and manitol, xylitol (choose only organic from birch trees—much of the xylitol on the market is made from by-products of the wood pulp industry or from cane pulp, seed hulls, or cornhusk), evaporated cane juice, cane sugar, sucanat, and molasses.

Artificial sweeteners. For the sake of your health, not just your weight, completely avoid all artificial sweeteners, which can cause a host of health problems. And if you think they're helping you lose weight, take a look at the research. People on sugar substitutes actually gain more weight than those using sugar.[35] And using sugar is a very bad choice for your weight as well as your health.

Check out the movie *Sweet Misery* for an eye-opening report on aspartame (NutraSweet). Dr. Woodrow C. Monte says, "Methanol [one of the breakdown products of aspartame] is considered a toxicant. The ingestion of two teaspoons is considered lethal in humans."[36] Long-term use can create a ticking time bomb for a large array of neurological illnesses, including (but not limited to) brain cancer, Lou Gehrig's disease, Graves' disease, chronic fatigue syndrome, multiple sclerosis (MS), and epilepsy.37

James Turner, chairman of Citizens for Health, has declared that the FDA should review their approval of Splenda based on a study of sucralose that reveals shocking new information about the potential harmful effects of this artificial sweetener on humans. Hundreds of consumers have complained about side effects from using Splenda. Turner went on to say that the study, published in the *Journal of Toxicology and Environmental Health*, confirms that the chemicals in the little yellow packets "should carry a big red warning label." According to a press release from the Citizens for health, the study found that "Splenda reduces the amount of good bacteria in the intestines by 50%, increases the pH level in the intestines, contributes to increases in body weight, and affects the P-glycoprotein (P-gp) in the body in such a way that crucial health-related drugs could be rejected."[38] The study is clear that this sweetener can also cause you to gain weight!

High-Fructose Corn Syrup Makes Your Brain Crave Food

The average American now consumes 145 pounds of high-fructose corn syrup per year (a corn sweetener found in most sodas and many processed foods). It's amazing everyone is not obese. New research proves exactly how high-fructose corn syrup bypasses normal energy balance systems in the body, causing the brain to want more food because it never really registers the calories of the high-fructose corn syrup.[39] There is also research indicating that high-fructose corn syrup turns on gene signaling that promotes fat formation and fat accumulation, which is likely to result in obesity, insulin resistance, and type 2 diabetes.[40]

Sweeteners to use sparingly include agave syrup, brown rice syrup, and pure maple syrup. I recommend stevia as the best sweetener to use.

Chapter 7

The Living Foods Menu Planner and Guide

If you fail to plan, you are planning to fail.
—Author unknown

HERE ARE TWO menu plans in this section—one for raw vegan and the other with a large percentage of the food raw but with some cooked foods and animal protein added. There is a reason for that. We are all different. It is true that one man's food is another man's poison. For example, some people absolutely thrive on raw fruit for breakfast. Most fruit makes me ill. It has too much sugar for me. I do well with vegetables, such as a green smoothie or vegetable juice with a lot of greens, but not fruit.

There are numerous individuals who got well eating strictly raw vegan cuisine. Others thrive on vegan diets that include cooked food. Notables like Dr. Neal Bernard, from The Physician's Committee for Responsible Medicine, and Dr. Dean Ornish, author of *Dr. Dean Ornish's Program for Reversing Heart Disease*, have confirmed the value of plant-based diets. My friend Paul Wenner, creator of the Gardenburger and the exciting new Gardenbar, healed his body early in life by becoming vegetarian. And my friend Vicki Chelf, author of *Vicki's Vegan Kitchen*, says she has never felt well eating muscle meats and thrives on a vegan diet.

But Dr. Joseph Mercola discovered quite the opposite. He says, "After finishing my family practice residency in 1985 I read the book *Fit for Life*, which encourages consumption of primarily raw fruits and vegetables. So I followed its recommendations and started eating fruit for breakfast. After a few weeks I had blood work done and was shocked to find my fasting triglycerides were nearly 3,000. Yes, three thousand...This was surprising because they had never been over 100 in the past. Clearly this diet was slowly killing me and I am convinced I would have died long ago had I remained on it. I now realize that the strict vegetarian or vegan approach probably helps some, but it was a disaster for me personally."[1]

Chris Masterjohn had a unique experience as well. He is one of many who have tried vegetarianism and eventually veganism in support of animal rights. He had hopes of attaining optimal health but ultimately failed to achieve this until taking a very different dietary approach. When he added red meat back into his diet, his panic attacks ceased within a few short weeks.[2]

As you can see, we're all different. Some thrive with muscle meats in their diet, while others thrive without any. However, no one needs a lot of meat, and meat eaters should consume only organic, grass-fed muscle meats. But we all need lots of vegetables. No one argues with that point. And the more veggies we consume raw, the more vibrantly healthy we become. If you want to glow with health, this is your path.

And everyone can do short-term "raw vegan weeks" for cleansing and detoxifying the system. It is particularly helpful after eating a lot of heavy food or overindulging. This was the practical wisdom of Lent—eating light in the spring after heavy winter foods. Also, a one- or two-day vegetable juice fast occasionally is very helpful for cleansing the body and gives your organs of elimination a rest.

The Fast Track One-Day Juice Diet

To accelerate weight loss or get a jump start on your health, try my One-Day Juice Diet or my Jump Start Weekend Weight-Loss Diet. I'll outline both programs for you before we get into the Living Foods Revolution Meal Plan.

For the One-Day Juice Diet you can pick a day you are off from work to make it more convenient for you, or you can juice ahead and take your juice to work. Some people like to have juice for dinner the night before and breakfast and lunch the next day, with a meal that evening. Choose what works for you.

This all-liquid day helps you detox your body and flush out fat. During this day you will drink only vegetable juice, vegetable broth, water, sparkling mineral water, and herbal, green, or white tea. Here's a sample plan to take you through the day.

Breakfast

- Green, white, or herbal tea with lemon juice or hot water with lemon and a dash of cayenne pepper (this helps the liver get moving)
- Vegetable juice of your choice

Midmorning

- 9:30 a.m.: 8 ounces of water or cranberry water
- 10:30 a.m.: Vegetable juice of choice
- 11:30 a.m.: Green, white, or herbal tea or 8 ounces of water or sparkling mineral water

NOTE: To make cranberry water, start with unsweetened cranberry juice—just juice, nothing added. Add 1–2 tablespoons of cranberry juice or cranberry concentrate to an 8-ounce glass of purified water. Adjust cranberry juice to taste. You may add a few drops of stevia as desired.

Lunch

- Vegetable juice recipe of choice

Midafternoon

- 1:30 p.m.: 8 ounces water, lemon water, or cranberry water
- 2:30 p.m.: 8 ounces water, lemon water, or cranberry water
- 3:00 p.m.: Vegetable juice of choice
- 4:00 p.m.: 8 ounces water, lemon water, or cranberry water
- 5:00 p.m.: 8 ounces water, lemon water, or cranberry water

Dinner

- Vegetable juice of choice (you may also add a cup of warm vegetable broth)
- Cup of herbal tea

NOTE: Sparkling mineral water may be substituted for water at any time. You may add a squeeze of lemon or lime or unsweetened cranberry juice for added flavor.

THE JUMP START WEEKEND WEIGHT-LOSS DIET

If you're doing the weekend jump start, start Friday evening with a juice or a green smoothie for dinner (there are some recipes for green smoothies in chapter 8), and follow the One-Day Juice Diet meal plan (outlined above) for Saturday and breakfast and lunch on Sunday. Then choose a raw food recipe for your Sunday dinner.

This is a great way to jump-start your living foods lifestyle, to jump-start a weight-loss program, or to lose a couple of pounds quickly to get ready for a special event.

If you find that you are too spacey or your blood sugar drops too low while on either the one-day or weekend liquid diets I've just described, add a bowl of raw energy soup such as Cherie's Yummy Energy Soup in *The Juice Lady's Turbo Diet* or a green smoothie for one meal. This liquid fast (some call it a "liquid feast"!) is a great boost to weight loss because it will especially help you get rid of stored-up water and toxins while at the same time rejuvenating your body.

The Juice Lady's Living Foods Revolution Meal Plan

DAY 1

Breakfast
- Juice of choice, such as Green Berry Blast (page 167) or Green Coconut Delight (page 189) with raw sunflower seeds
- Green, white, or herbal tea (and a squeeze of lemon is nice)

Midmorning snack
- Juice of choice, herbal tea, or cranberry water
- Granny Smith or pippin apple or 2 tablespoons of raw seeds or nuts

Lunch
- Walnut Zucchini Greens (page 196) or salad of choice
- 2–3 Awesome Corn Crackers (page 207)

Midafternoon snack
- Juice of choice, herbal tea, or cranberry water
- Veggie sticks

Dinner
- Juice of choice, such as You Are Loved Cocktail (page 162)
- Dinner salad with Sesame Dressing (page 199)
- Cherie's Nut Burgers (page 209) with Healthy Raw Ketchup (page 200)
- Raw Zucchini Noodles (page 212) with olive oil, garlic, and basil

DAY 2

Breakfast
- Juice of choice, such as Fresh Pink Morning (page 163)
- Buckwheat Granola (page 195) with almond, oat, or rice milk
- Green, white, or herbal tea (and a squeeze of lemon is nice)

Midmorning snack
- Juice of choice, herbal tea, or cranberry water
- Veggie sticks

Lunch
- Borscht in the Raw (page 192)
- Dr. Nina's Russian Cabbage Slaw (page 197)

Midafternoon snack
- Juice of choice (optional)
- Spicy Kale Chips (page 204)

Dinner
- Juice of choice, such as Tomato and Spice (page 160)
- Chef Avi Dalene's Green Tortillas (page 211) with Nan's Sunflower Pate (page 213) and tomato salsa
- Green salad with Creamy Green Dressing (page 200)

DAY 3

Breakfast
- Juice of choice, such as Happy-Mood Morning (page 175)
- Apple Muesli (page 195)
- Green, white, or herbal tea (and a squeeze of lemon is nice)

Midmorning snack
- Juice of choice, herbal tea, or cranberry water
- Half dozen sun-dried or naturally processed green or black organic olives

Lunch
- Mock "Salmon" Pate (page 213) with Raw Almond Mayo (page 203)
- 2–3 Flax Crackers (page 205)

Midafternoon snack

- Juice of choice or cranberry water
- Veggie sticks with 1 tablespoon raw almond butter

Dinner

- Juice of choice, such as The Ginger Hopper With a Twist (page 163)
- Almond Roulade (page 214)
- Marinated Collard Greens (page 214)

DAY 4

Breakfast

- Juice of choice, such as Cranberry-Pear Fat Buster (page 172)
- Nutty Delight (page 192)
- Green, white, or herbal tea (and a squeeze of lemon is nice)

Midmorning snack

- Juice of choice, herbal tea, or cranberry water
- 12 raw almonds

Lunch

- Red Bell Pepper Soup (page 193)
- Sliced tomatoes with extra-virgin olive oil and balsamic vinegar
- 2–3 Veggie Nut Crackers (page 206)

Midafternoon snack

- Juice of choice, herbal tea, or cranberry water
- Piece of low-sugar fruit such as a green apple

Dinner

- Juice of choice, such as Goin' Green (page 169)
- Sliced cucumbers with balsamic vinegar
- Raw Zucchini Noodles With Marinara Sauce (page 212)

DAY 5

Breakfast

- Juice of choice, such as The Morning Energizer (page 174)

- Lemon Muesli (page 196) with oat, almond, or rice milk
- Green, white, or herbal tea (and a squeeze of lemon is nice)

Midmorning snack
- Juice of choice, herbal tea, or cranberry water
- 2 tablespoons raw sunflower seeds

Lunch
- Winter Salad (page 197)
- 1–2 Nan's Carrot Curry Flax Krax (page 206)

Midafternoon snack
- Juice of choice, herbal tea, or cranberry water
- 2 tablespoons raw sunflower seeds

Dinner
- Juice of choice, such as Peppy Parsley (page 175)
- Mexican Almond Dip (page 203)
- 2–3 Awesome Corn Crackers (page 207)
- Chef Avi Dalene's Green Tortillas (page 211) and Nan's Sunflower Pate (page 213) with Mango Salsa (page 215) or tomato salsa

DAY 6

Breakfast
- Juice of choice, such as Happy-Mood Morning (page 174)
- Sprouted Buckwheat Groats (page 196) with milk of choice and ground nuts or raw seeds
- Green, white, or herbal tea (and a squeeze of lemon is nice)

Midmorning snack
- Juice of choice, herbal tea, or cranberry water
- Granny Smith or pippin apple or veggie sticks

Lunch
- Sprouted Quinoa Salad (page 198)
- 2–3 Veggie Nut Crackers (page 206)

Midafternoon snack
- Juice of choice, herbal tea, or cranberry water
- 6 raw almonds

Dinner

- Juice of choice, such as Green Lemonade (page 167)
- Gourmet Pesto Pizza (page 212)
- Sliced tomatoes with extra-virgin olive oil and balsamic vinegar

DAY 7

Breakfast

- Juice of choice, such as Weight-Loss Buddy (page 172)
- Kale-Pear Smoothie (page 189)
- Green, white, or herbal tea (and a squeeze of lemon is nice)

Midmorning snack

- Juice of choice, herbal tea, or cranberry water
- Zucchini Hummus (page 215) with 2 Awesome Corn Crackers (page 207)

Lunch

- Almond Falafel (page 214) with Sunflower Dill Sauce (page 198)
- Icy Spicy Gazpacho (page 193)

Midafternoon snack

- Juice of choice, herbal tea, or cranberry water
- 1 Granny Smith or pippin apple

Dinner

- Juice of choice, such as Raging Beet-Jalapeño (page 175)
- Sunny Delight Enchiladas With Corn Tortillas (page 210) and Mango Salsa (page 215)
- Green salad with dressing of choice

Menu Plan With Some Cooked Vegan Foods and Animal Products, as Desired

DAY 1

Breakfast

- Juice of choice, such as Green Berry Blast (page 167) and/or
- Green Coconut Delight with raw sunflower seeds (page 189)

- Green, white, or herbal tea (and a squeeze of lemon is nice)

Midmorning snack
- Juice of choice, herbal tea, or cranberry water
- Boiled egg or 2 tablespoons of raw seeds or nuts

Lunch
- Caesar Salad (with option of chicken strips or broiled salmon)
- 1–2 Awesome Corn Crackers (page 207)

Midafternoon snack
- Juice of choice, herbal tea, or cranberry water
- Veggie sticks

Dinner
- Juice of choice, such as You Are Loved Cocktail (page 162)
- Dinner salad with Sesame Dressing (page 199)
- Carrot Sauce With Asparagus and Fresh Peas Over Rice (page 218)

DAY 2

Breakfast
- Juice of choice, such as Fresh Pink Morning (page 163)
- Buckwheat Granola (page 195) or old-fashioned oatmeal with almond, oat, or rice milk
- Green, white, or herbal tea (and a squeeze of lemon is nice)

Midmorning snack
- Juice of choice, herbal tea, or cranberry water
- Veggie sticks

Lunch
- Borscht in the Raw (page 192) or bean or vegetable soup (cooked)
- Dr. Nina's Russian Cabbage Slaw (page 197)

Midafternoon snack
- Juice of choice, herbal tea, or cranberry water
- Spicy Kale Chips (page 204)

Dinner

- Juice of choice, such as Tomato and Spice (page 160)
- Stir-fry with brown and wild rice
- Green salad with Ginger-Lime Dressing (page 199)

DAY 3

Breakfast

- Juice of choice, such as Happy-Mood Morning (page 174)
- Apple Muesli (page 195)
- Green, white, or herbal tea (and a squeeze of lemon is nice)

Midmorning snack

- Juice of choice, herbal tea, or cranberry water
- Half dozen sun-dried or naturally processed green or black organic olives

Lunch

- Main course salad of choice with cup of chili or soup of choice
- 2–3 Flax Crackers (page 205)

Midafternoon snack

- Juice of choice, herbal tea, or cranberry water
- Veggie sticks with 1 tablespoon raw almond butter

Dinner

- Juice of choice, such as The Ginger Hopper With a Twist (page 163)
- Squash and Arugula Enchiladas (page 217)
- Marinated Collard Greens (page 214)

DAY 4

Breakfast

- Juice of choice, such as Cranberry-Pear Fat Buster (page 172)
- Nutty Delight (page 192)
- Green, white, or herbal tea (and a squeeze of lemon is nice)

Midmorning snack
- Juice of choice or herbal tea
- 12 raw almonds

Lunch
- Red Bell Pepper Soup (page 193) or salad of choice
- Sliced tomatoes with extra-virgin olive oil and balsamic vinegar
- 1 Veggie Nut Cracker (page 206)

Midafternoon snack
- Juice of choice, herbal tea, or cranberry water
- Piece of low-sugar fruit such as a green apple

Dinner
- Juice of choice, such as Goin' Green (page 169)
- Sliced cucumbers with balsamic vinegar
- Vegan dish of choice or baked chicken, fish, or turkey

DAY 5

Breakfast
- Juice of choice, such as The Morning Energizer (page 174)
- Lemon Muesli (page 196) with oat, almond, or rice milk
- Green, white, or herbal tea (and a squeeze of lemon is nice)

Midmorning snack
- Juice of choice or herbal tea
- 2 tablespoons raw sunflower seeds

Lunch
- Winter Salad (page 197)
- 1 Nan's Carrot Curry Flax Krax (page 206)

Midafternoon snack
- Juice of choice, herbal tea, or cranberry water
- 2 tablespoons raw sunflower seeds

Dinner

- Juice of choice, such as Peppy Parsley (page 175)
- Mexican Almond Dip (page 203)
- 2–3 Awesome Corn Crackers (page 207)
- Chef Avi Dalene's Green Tortillas (page 211) and Nan's Sunflower Pate (page 213) with Mango Salsa (page 215) or tomato salsa

DAY 6

Breakfast

- Juice of choice, such as Happy-Mood Morning (page 174)
- Sprouted Buckwheat Groats (page 196) with milk of choice and ground nuts or raw seeds
- Green, white, or herbal tea (and a squeeze of lemon is nice)

Midmorning snack

- Juice of choice, herbal tea, or cranberry water
- Boiled egg or veggie sticks

Lunch

- Nicole's Butternut Squash Soup (page 219)
- 2–3 Veggie Nut Crackers (page 206)

Midafternoon snack

- Juice of choice, herbal tea, or cranberry water
- 6 raw almonds

Dinner

- Juice of choice, such as Green Lemonade (page 167)
- Lentil-Spinach Skillet Dinner (page 219)
- Sliced tomatoes with extra-virgin olive oil and balsamic vinegar

DAY 7

Breakfast

- Juice of choice, such as Weight-Loss Buddy (page 172) or
- Kale-Pear Smoothie (page 189) and/or
- Bowl of old-fashioned oatmeal with milk of choice
- Green, white, or herbal tea (and a squeeze of lemon is nice)

Midmorning snack
- Juice of choice, herbal tea, or cranberry water
- Dehydrated tomato slices

Lunch
- Almond Falafel (page 214) with Sunflower Dill Sauce (page 198)
- Icy Spicy Gazpacho (page 193)

Midafternoon snack
- Juice of choice, herbal tea, or cranberry water
- 1 Granny Smith or pippin apple

Dinner
- Juice of choice, such as Raging Beet-Jalapeño (page 175)
- Caesar salad
- Nicole's Stuffed Acorn Squash (page 219)

The Best Way to Cook Your Food

Though this is a book about living foods, unless you go all raw vegan, as some people have, you'll want to cook or warm up leftovers in the healthiest way possible. How you do that is extremely important to your health. That's why I'm recommending that you only use your stovetop, oven, toaster oven, countertop grill, or convection oven. I think when you finish reading the data I've collected, you'll want to toss out your microwave for good reasons.

It has been found that radiation exposure can weaken the immune system and cause health-related problems such as cancer and degenerative diseases. It may also cause ailments such as "persistent cough, headaches, sleep disturbances, and gastrointestinal dysfunction," notes Dr. J. D. Decuypere. She has observed that respiratory illnesses such as asthma, bronchitis, chronic cough, and allergies have been increasing since the late 1970s, which prompted her to do her own investigation on radiation in our food.[3]

Though there are numerous ways that we are exposed to radiation, there are two ways that it enters our food—microwave ovens and irradiation of food. Radiating food in a microwave oven is convenient, and many people use their microwave daily. But studies have shown that it may negatively impact the nutrition of the food, and it may be harmful to the people who eat it.

The British medical journal *The Lancet* (December 9, 1989) reported that when microwaving baby bottles, "one of the amino acids, L-proline, was converted to its d-isomer, which is known to be neurotoxic ([poisonous to the] nervous system) and nephrotoxic ([poisonous to the] kidneys). It's bad enough that many babies are not nursed. Now they are given fake milk (baby formula) made even more toxic by microwaving."[4]

The radiation process of a microwave oven can alter a food's molecular structure and create new chemicals called unique radiolytic products (URPs). If that sounds harmless to you, then you need to know that URPs include benzene, formaldehyde, and a host of mutagens and carcinogens—a fact that should alert you to the potential hazards of eating microwaved foods.[5]

A study performed by Dr. Hans Hertel of Switzerland found that food prepared in microwave ovens had molecular alteration, but he found too that it also altered the blood chemistry of people eating it. Volunteers had:

- Altered hemoglobin and cholesterol values, especially HDL and LDL values and ratio
- Lymphocytes (white blood cells) that demonstrated a distinct short-term decrease following consumption of microwaved food than after eating anything else

Dr. Hertel said these changes point toward degeneration of health. The natural repair mechanisms of cells become disturbed, which forces cells to respond to a "state-of-emergency" energy supply, exchanging aerobic (oxygen-based) for anaerobic (no oxygen) respiration. This constitutes a cancer-type effect on the blood—cancer cells are anaerobic.[6]

Here are some of the results of various studies on microwaving foods:

- Creation of d-Nitrosodiethanolamines—a cancer-causing agent
- Creation of cancer-causing agents within protein compounds in milk and cereal grains
- Alteration in the breakdown of glucoside and galactoside elements within frozen fruits when thawed in a microwave oven
- Altered catabolic behavior of plant alkaloids when raw, cooked, or frozen vegetables were microwave heated for even a short time
- Cancer-causing free radicals formed within certain trace-mineral molecular formations in plants, especially in raw root vegetables
- A higher percentage of cancerous cells in the blood

- Malfunctions occurring in the lymphatic system, causing degeneration of the immune system's capacity to protect itself against cancerous growth
- Altered food substances leading to disorders in the digestive system
- A statistically higher incidence of stomach and intestinal cancers, plus a general degeneration of peripheral cellular tissues with a gradual breakdown of digestive and excretory system function
- Significant decrease in the nutritional value of all foods studied
- A decrease in the availability of B-complex vitamins, vitamin C, vitamin E, essential minerals, and lipotropic nutrients
- Destruction of the nutritional value of protein in meat
- Lowering of the metabolic activity of alkaloids, glucosides, galactosides and nitrilosides (basic plant substances in fruits and vegetables)
- Marked acceleration of structural disintegration in all foods[7]

Microwaving food in plastic containers poses an additional risk of the food absorbing dangerous chemicals released from the plastic when it is heated.

While the dangers of using microwave ovens are still embroiled in battle and controversy, it is highly recommended that you not use a microwave at all—even for heating water. Recently a friend sent an e-mail to me about a woman who conducted a home experiment with two similar plants. She watered one with cooled microwaved water and the other with tap water. The microwave-watered plant died rather quickly.

SET YOUR GOALS

In getting started, it's important to keep track of the foods you eat each day. At the end of this chapter is a daily food diary; you can make copies of this diary and fill it out each day. Write down everything you eat. Sometimes we don't realize all the stuff we are eating until we write it down, because we take a bite of something and forget about it, or we grab a few nuts or a couple of candies from someone's desk at work, pop them in our mouths, and off we go! Or we may get a snack from a vending machine at break. It's the small things that add up fast and often derail us from our healthy lifestyle path.

That's why it's important to note everything you eat so you can make changes that are helpful to achieve your goals. Every day take inventory. Are you drinking the water you need for optimal health, which is eight glasses a day? How about green or white tea, which has thermogenic effects? Are you drinking two glasses of vegetable juice each day? Are you often drinking green juices? What food choices did you make during the day? Were at least half to three-fourths of the foods you ate raw? How much food did you eat in the evening? If you look at what you're doing objectively, you can make adjustments that will move you forward.

There's a quote I read often: "To get something you never had, you have to do something you've never done." You know what they say about the people who keep doing the same thing over and over again and expect different results—that's insanity! One definition of insanity is extreme foolishness. To become a new you, you must see yourself in a new way—as the person you choose to become—and adopt new action steps. You will succeed by choosing outcome-based behaviors you haven't done consistently before.

This book is about a living foods lifestyle revolution—a revolution in your life. As you set your goals, it's helpful to reframe your thinking. You can do this. You can make the changes necessary to live a vibrantly healthy life.

Start a goal-minded picture board. Cut out a picture of a person that resembles the healthy person you want to be. Put it up in a place where you can see it often. You may be wondering if this stuff could possibly work.

It did for me. I made a storyboard of pictures years ago when I set my career goals. I still display it in my office. I had a picture of a writer on the page with a goal of writing many books. At the time I had only cowritten one book. This book, *The Juice Lady's Living Foods Revolution*, is number eighteen. I put a picture of a television in one corner because I wanted to combine my field of speech communications (that was my undergrad degree) with my master's degree in nutrition. To date, I've appeared in six infomercials and have appeared for thirteen years on QVC, where I often sold one million dollars in product per show. I have a ship on that board because I wanted to be a speaker on cruises. Last fall was our maiden voyage for our first (and very successful I might add) "Health & Fitness Cruise" to Mexico. Next year it's the Caribbean.

In 1995 I met George Foreman at the Gourmet Products Show in Las

Vegas. He was there for a fight. I was there for the Salton Housewares booth with the Juiceman juicer. At the same time, Salton was rolling out the Lean, Mean, Fat-Reducing Grilling Machine. When I met George at the show, I decided I wanted to work with him and the grill. I got an autographed picture and put it on my bulletin board in my office. Every day, whenever I looked at his picture, I'd say, "I'm going to work with you."

To date, I've coauthored a book with George—*Knock Out the Fat Barbecue & Grilling Cookbook*, and I've appeared in three of the grilling infomercials. I have appeared with the grill for thirteen years on QVC in the United States, London, and Germany. For a number of the key shows I appeared with George. I got more than I'd planned on.

As you set your goals, tack up your storyboard where you can see it. What are your goals? Weight loss? More energy? Better sleep, mood, or stamina? Health improvement? Bodybuilding? What is your purpose in life? What gives you excitement and energy for living? If you don't know your purpose, why you're here on this earth, you may not garner the willpower to make the right choices day in and day out. As you embark on your healthy lifestyle journey, keep a positive mental attitude. Tell yourself each day that you can do this. You can achieve your goals. Praise yourself often for all the right choices you make. Don't beat yourself up for the mistakes. You can become a new you. You can fulfill the purpose for your life in the trim, fit body that will best help you run your unique race of life.

I'm in your corner cheering for you. My prayers are with you. I'd love to hear your story—your small successes and your great ones. Don't ever give up. Remember it's worth it to hang in there, even if it's one day at a time as it was for me in the past. Through all the obstacles, tragedies, and trials you may have experienced, you've kept going. You're here reading this book. I applaud you for that. One day you'll be standing in your dream. You can do it! One day, just like so many other people I've worked with, you will be living your life to the fullest because with a healthy body and a healthy mind, you can live your purpose to the fullest.

Daily Food Diary for the Juice Lady's Living Foods Revolution Diet

Day _____

Vegetable juice and other liquids

- Glass 1 _____
- Glass 2 _____
- Water (minimum eight 8-ounce glasses per day)

  _____
- Herbal tea _____
- Green tea _____

Supplements

- _____
- _____

Foods

- Grains _____
- Vegetables _____
- Fruit _____
- Meat/fish/poultry _____
- Fats _____
- Other _____

DIET DIARY

Breakfast	
Midmorning snack	
Lunch	
Midafternoon snack	
Dinner	

Chapter 8

The Living Foods Recipes

When you sit to dine with a ruler...do not crave his delicacies, for that food is deceptive.
—Proverbs 23:1–3, niv

A s the proverb says, rich foods are deceptive. We want more and more of these foods, but they never seem to satisfy the body. Many packaged items are addictive, purposely designed that way so we'll eat more of them. Living foods and whole foods recipes, though not rich with the fare that contributes to ill health, are far more satisfying. We can eat a normal portion and feel like we've had all we want. And the good news is that they also taste delicious. These foods will nurture both your body and soul. The recipes in this chapter are among my favorites. I hope you enjoy them too.

Juice Recipes

The juice recipes in this chapter use more vegetables than fruit, and the fruits and vegetables are mostly low glycemic. You may change any of the recipes to fit your needs. If there is something you are allergic to in a recipe, omit it or substitute another food. If you are diabetic, prediabetic, hypoglycemic, have a problem with yeast, or have cancer, you may need to omit almost all fruit, with the exception of lemons and limes. And lemon is a nice addition to almost any recipe; it's also very alkaline. Cranberries are also very low in sugar. All other berries and green apples are next in line as the lowest sugar fruits.

I've grouped juice recipes into sections with nutrition information about many of them so you could find the juice combinations that best meet your goals.

General Recipes for Vibrant Health

Tomato and Spice

2 medium tomatoes
2 dark green leaves
2 radishes
Small handful parsley
1 lime or lemon, peeled if not organic
Dash of hot sauce

Cut produce to fit your juicer's feed tube. Juice all ingredients and stir. Pour into a glass and drink as soon as possible. Serves 1.

Refreshing Mint Cocktail

2 stalks fennel with leaves
1 cucumber, peeled if not organic
1 stalk celery
1 green apple such as Granny Smith or pippin
1 handful mint
1-inch-chunk ginger root

Cut produce to fit your juicer's feed tube. Juice all ingredients and stir. Pour into a glass and drink as soon as possible. Serves 1-2.

Beet, Carrot, Coconut Blast

4-5 carrots, scrubbed well, tops removed, ends trimmed
1 small beet with leaves
½-1 cup coconut milk
Dash cayenne pepper

Juice the carrots and beets. Pour into a glass and add the coconut milk and cayenne pepper. Stir. Drink as soon as possible. Serves 2.

Jicama Delight

2-inch by 4- or 5-inch chunk of jicama, scrubbed well or peeled
½ green apple
½ cucumber, peeled if not organic
¼ daikon radish, trimmed and scrubbed
1-inch-chunk ginger root, scrubbed, peeled if old
½ lemon or lime, peeled if not organic

Cut produce to fit your juicer's feed tube. Juice all ingredients and stir. Pour into a glass and drink as soon as possible. Serves 1.

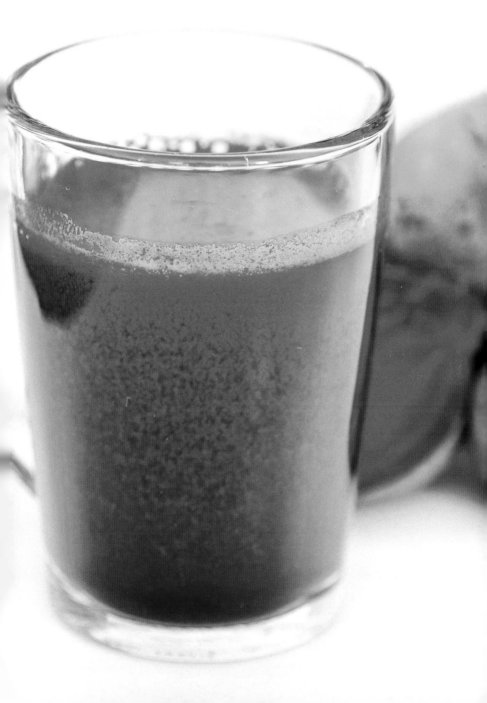

Radish Surprise

5 carrots, scrubbed well, green tops removed, ends trimmed
1 cucumber, peeled if not organic, or 1 large chunk of jicama
5–6 radishes
1 lemon, peeled if not organic

Cut produce to fit your juicer's feed tube. Juice all ingredients and stir. Pour into a glass. Serve at room temperature or chilled, as desired. Serves 1.

Root Veggie Medley

3–4 carrots, scrubbed well, tops removed, ends trimmed
1 cucumber, peeled if not organic
½ beet, scrubbed well, with stems and leaves
½–1 small kohlrabi, with leaves
1 lemon, peeled if not organic
½ apple (green has less sugar)
1-inch-chunk ginger root, peeled

Cut produce to fit your juicer's feed tube. Juice all ingredients and stir. Pour into a glass and drink as soon as possible. Serves 1–2.

South of the Border Cocktail

1 medium tomato
1 cucumber, peeled if not organic
1 handful cilantro
1 lime, peeled if not organic
Dash of hot sauce (optional)

Cut produce to fit your juicer's feed tube. Juice all ingredients and stir. Pour into a glass and drink as soon as possible. Serves 1.

You Are Loved Cocktail

3 carrots, scrubbed well, tops removed, ends trimmed
2 celery stalks, with leaves
1 cucumber, peeled if not organic
1 handful spinach
1 lemon, peeled if not organic
½ beet, scrubbed well, with stems and leaves

Cut produce to fit your juicer's feed tube. Juice all ingredients and stir. Pour into a glass and drink as soon as possible. Serves 1–2.

Springtime Tonic

Asparagus is a natural diuretic, which helps flush toxins from the body and promotes kidney cleansing. It's a great tonic for the kidneys. This recipe is a great way to use up asparagus stems.

1 tomato
1 cucumber, peeled if not organic
8 asparagus stems
Handful wild greens
1 lemon, peeled if not organic

Cut produce to fit your juicer's feed tube. Juice all ingredients and stir. Pour into a glass and drink as soon as possible. Serves 1–2.

The Ginger Hopper With a Twist

5 medium carrots, scrubbed well, green tops removed, ends trimmed
1 green apple
1-inch-chunk fresh ginger root, peeled
½ lemon, peeled if not organic

Cut produce to fit your juicer's feed tube. Juice all ingredients and stir. Pour into a glass and drink as soon as possible. Serves 1.

Fresh Pink Morning

1 large pink grapefruit, peeled
½ green apple
1-inch-chunk fresh ginger root, peeled

Cut produce to fit your juicer's feed tube. Juice all ingredients and stir. Pour into a glass and drink as soon as possible. Serves 1.

Tomato Florentine

2 tomatoes
4–5 sprigs basil
1 large handful spinach
1 lemon, peeled if not organic

Juice one tomato. Wrap the basil in several spinach leaves. Turn off the machine and add the spinach and basil. Turn the machine back on and gently tap to juice them. Juice the remaining tomato and lemon. Stir juice, pour into a glass and drink as soon as possible. Serves 1.

Veggie Time Cocktail

4 carrots, scrubbed well, green tops removed, ends trimmed
1 handful rapini or other dark greens
1 lemon, peeled if not organic
2-inch chunk jicama, scrubbed or peeled if not organic
1 handful watercress
1 garlic clove

Cut produce to fit your juicer's feed tube. Juice all ingredients and stir. Pour into a glass and drink as soon as possible. Serves 1–2.

Waldorf Twist

1 green apple
3 stalks organic celery with leaves
1 lemon, peeled if not organic

Cut produce to fit your juicer's feed tube. Juice all ingredients and stir. Pour into a glass and drink as soon as possible. Serves 1.

Green Juices

There are many greens that can be juiced, such as collard leaves, Swiss chard, beet tops, kale, kohlrabi leaves, mustard greens, parsley, spinach, lettuce, cilantro, arugula, rapini, and dandelion greens. All you need is a juicer and some yummy recipes, and you can easily consume a couple of fistsful of greens every day.

It is believed that our ancient ancestors ate up to 6 pounds of green leaves per day, when in season. Probably they walked from one place to another, just picking and eating leaves as they went. Can you imagine eating a grocery bag full of greens each day when they are in season? Few of us even eat the minimum USDA recommendation of five servings of vegetables and fruit a day or 3 cups of dark green vegetables per week. And yet, these veggies deliver a bonanza of vitamins, minerals, enzymes, biophotons, and phytonutrients.

Calorie for calorie, dark green leafy vegetables are among the most concentrated source of nutrition of any food—and with the least calories. They are a rich source of minerals, including iron, calcium, potassium, and magnesium, plus vitamins K, C, and E, along with many of the B vitamins. They also provide a variety of phytonutrients, including beta-carotene, lutein, and zeaxanthin, which protect our cells from damage and our eyes from age-related diseases. Dark green leaves also contain small amounts of omega-3 fats. All this makes dark greens one of the best choices you can make in your diet. So juice them on a regular basis.

Bitter greens

It is believed that bitters support the heart, small intestines, kidneys, and liver, as well as reduce fever. They offer us four tastes—sweet, salty, bitter, and sour—with bitter now gaining culinary respect. They should be a part of our choices for juicing as well as our cooking creations.

The following primer on bitter greens should help you with choosing flavors that combine well with other vegetables and fruit.

- Arugula—green or red, oak-shaped leaf; nutty, peppery, hot and sharp
- Beet greens—purple-red veins and bright green flesh on the leaves; very tangy with a hint of mustard and beet

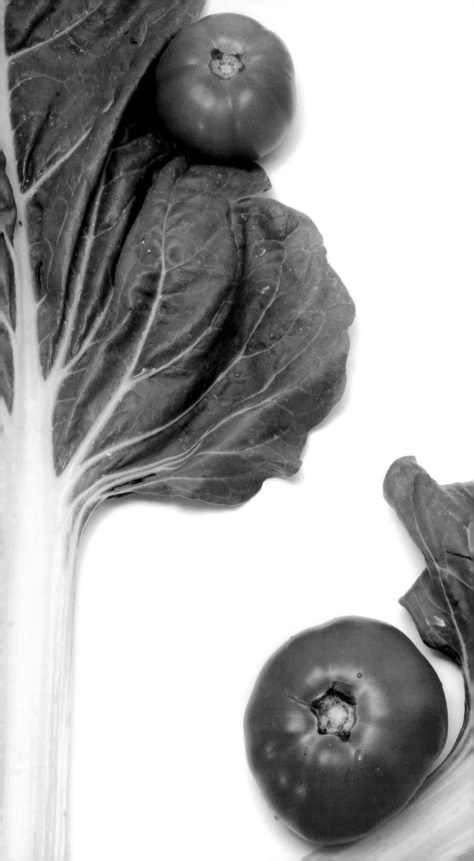

- Cress—watercress is widely available; the taste is hot, sharp, and biting
- Endive—long, narrow, leaves, white at the base and pale yellow-green at the tips; bitter
- Frisee—stiff, short, skinny leaves with curly edges; may be green or blanched with white stems and yellow-green tips; mild, slightly bitter flavor
- Kale—large deep green leaves, curled at the edges; resembles broccoli in flavor but with a peppery, bitter finish
- Mustards—red or green leaves; sharp, pungent with a hint of hot mustard and horseradish flavor
- Nasturtium—round, disk-shaped leaves and bright yellow-red-orange flowers; hot, peppery taste with a hint of horseradish
- Sorrel—long oval shape; piquant, tart, and tangy with a citrus overtone; once considered to be poisonous due to its taste
- Swiss chard—broad, fan-shaped green leaf, wide white stems and veins (some have red or yellow veins); mildly bitter
- Tatsoi—round, deep green, waxy leaves; zippy, slightly bitter taste

Green Berry Blast

1 cucumber, peeled if not organic
4 dark green leaves such as collard, chard, or kale
1 cup blueberries (if frozen, thaw first)
1 apple (green is lower in sugar)
½ lemon, peeled if not organic

Cut produce to fit your juicer's feed tube. Juice half of the cucumber. Roll the green leaves and push through the juicer with other half of the cucumber. Turn off the machine and pour in the berries, then place the plunger on top. Turn the machine on and push the berries through. Add the apple and lemon, and juice. Stir the juice and drink as soon as possible. Serves 2.

Green Lemonade

2 apples (green is lower in sugar)
½ lemon, peeled if not organic
1 handful of your favorite greens

Cut produce to fit your juicer's feed tube. Juice all ingredients and stir. Pour into a glass and drink as soon as possible. Serves 1.

Super Green Sprout Drink

Avoid alfalfa sprouts. Alfalfa is becoming one of the top GMO crops in the nation.

1 cucumber, peeled if not organic
1 stalk celery with leaves, as desired
1 small handful sprouts such as broccoli or radish
1 large handful sunflower sprouts
1 small handful buckwheat sprouts
1 lemon, peeled if not organic

Cut produce to fit your juicer's feed tube. Juice all ingredients and stir. Pour into a glass and drink as soon as possible. Serves 1.

Green Recharger

1 cucumber, peeled if not organic
1 handful sunflower sprouts
1 handful buckwheat sprouts
1 small handful clover sprouts
1 kale leaf
1 large handful spinach
1 lime, peeled if not organic

Cut the cucumber to fit your juicer's feed tube. Juice half of the cucumber first. Bunch up the sprouts and wrap in the kale leaf. Turn off the machine and add them. Turn the machine back on and tap with the rest of the cucumber to gently push the sprouts and kale through followed by spinach. Then juice the remaining cucumber and lime. Stir ingredients, pour into a glass, and drink as soon as possible. Serves 1–2.

Green Delight

2 Swiss chard leaves
1 celery stalk
1 handful spinach
1 handful parsley
1 apple (green is lower in sugar)
½ lemon, peeled if not organic

Cut produce to fit your juicer's feed tube. Roll the chard leaves and push through the juicer with the celery stalk. Add the spinach and parsley and push through juicer with the apple and lemon. Stir the juice and drink as soon as possible. Serves 1.

Wild Green Energy Cocktail

Wild greens reduce the desire for starchy foods, thus making them an excellent weight-loss helper.

1 cucumber, peeled if not organic
1 celery stalk
1 handful wild greens such as dandelion, nettles, plantain,
    lamb's quarters, or sorrel
1 apple (green is lower in sugar)
1 lemon, peeled if not organic

Cut all ingredients to fit your juicer's feed tube. Juice all ingredients and stir. Pour into a glass and drink as soon as possible. Serves 1.

3 K-Green Cocktail

2-3 kohlrabi leaves
1 kale leaf
1 kiwi fruit
1 celery stalk
1 apple (green has less sugar)
½ lemon, peeled if not organic

Cut produce to fit your juicer's feed tube. Roll the leaves and push through the juicer with the kiwi fruit and celery stalk. Add the apple and lemon, then juice. Stir the juice and drink as soon as possible. Serves 1.

Greens of Life

2 chard leaves
2 collard leaves
1 handful parsley
1 cucumber, peeled if not organic
1 lemon, peeled if not organic

Roll leaves, place parsley inside one leaf, and push through juicer with cucumber, followed by the lemon. Stir the juice and drink as soon as possible. Serves 1-2.

Goin' Green

Several beet leaves
Several kohlrabi leaves
2 stalks celery
1 cucumber, peeled if not organic
3 carrots
1 pear
½ lemon, peeled if not organic

Place some green leaves in your juicer; alternate leaves with celery followed by cucumber, carrot, pear, and lemon. Stir the juice and drink as soon as possible. Serves 1-2.

Arugula Cocktail

Pound for pound arugula is one of *the most* potent anticancer foods. Some of its phytochemicals, such as glucosinolate and sulforaphane, are responsible for stimulating enzymes that help the body cleanse away toxins and carcinogens. It also contains carotenes that can protect against sun damage, heart disease, and cancer. In addition, these nutrients improve communication between cells, something that may play a large role in healthy cellular function.

> 1 cucumber, peeled if not organic
> 1 handful arugula
> 2 stalks celery
> 1-inch-chunk ginger root
> 1 lemon, peeled if not organic

Cut cucumber in half. Juice one-half cucumber. Bunch up arugula and push through juicer with other half of the cucumber, followed by celery, ginger root, and lemon. Stir the juice and drink as soon as possible. Serves 1.

Mustard Surprise

Mustard greens provide what's known as "hot energy" in Chinese medicine. It promotes good circulation and relieves congestion.

> 3 carrots, scrubbed well, tops removed, ends trimmed
> 2 stalks celery
> 2-3 mustard leaves
> 1 cucumber, peeled if not organic
> 1 apple (green is lower in sugar)

Juice carrots and celery, roll mustard leaves and place in juicer. Push the greens through with the cucumber and apple. Stir the juice and drink as soon as possible. Serves 1-2.

Wheatgrass Light

Wheatgrass is loaded with chlorophyll and a "boatload" of nutrients. It provides one of the healthiest juices you could drink.

> 1 green apple, washed
> 1 handful wheatgrass, rinsed
> ½ lemon, peeled if not organic
> 2-3 sprigs mint, rinsed (optional)

Cut produce to fit your juicer's feed tube. Starting with apple, juice all ingredients and stir. Pour into a glass and drink as soon as possible. Serves 1.

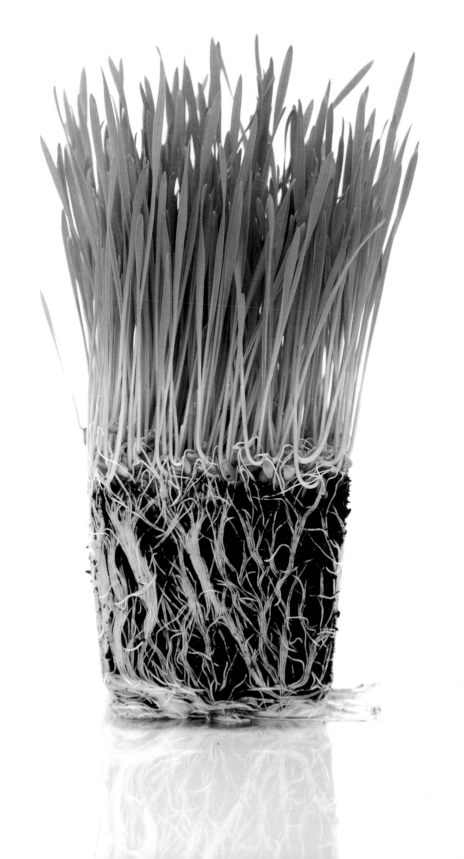

Wheatgrass With Coconut Water

1–2 oz. wheatgrass juice
8 oz. coconut water

Pour wheatgrass juice into a glass. Add coconut water and stir. Serves 1.

Weight-Loss Recipes

Cranberry-Pear Fat Blaster

Studies show that cranberries boost metabolism and their acids help dissolve fat. In addition, cranberries are a diuretic, which helps you get rid of stored up water. They also have soluble fiber, which is not lost entirely with juicing.

2 pears, Bartlett or Asian
½ cucumber, peeled if not organic
¼ lemon, peeled if not organic
2 Tbsp. cranberries, fresh or thawed if frozen
½- to 1-inch-chunk ginger root

Cut produce to fit your juicer's feed tube. Juice all ingredients and stir. Pour into a glass and drink as soon as possible. Serves 1–2.

Weight-Loss Buddy

Jerusalem artichoke juice combined with carrot and beet is a traditional remedy for satisfying cravings for sweets and junk food. The key is to sip it slowly when you get a craving for high-fat or high-carb foods.

3–4 carrots, scrubbed well, tops removed, ends trimmed
1 Jerusalem artichoke, scrubbed well
1 cucumber, peeled if not organic
1 lemon, peeled if not organic
½ small beet, scrubbed well, with stems and leaves

Cut produce to fit your juicer's feed tube. Juice all ingredients and stir. Pour into a glass and drink as soon as possible. Serves 1–2.

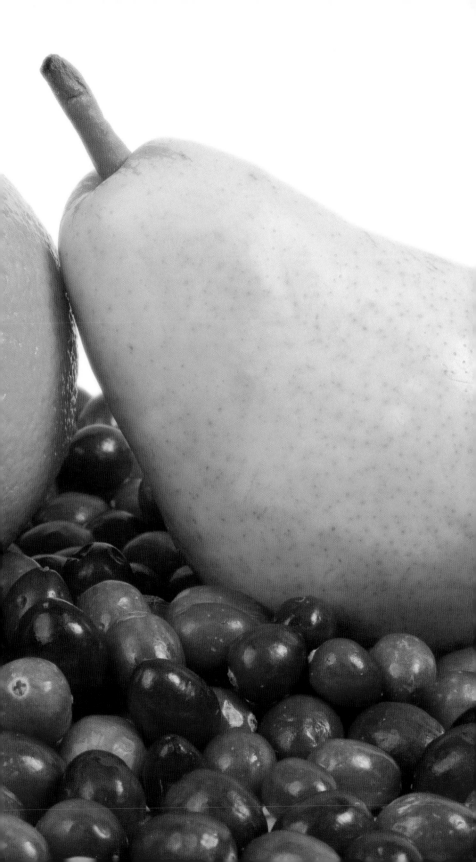

Energizing Cocktails

All the juice recipes in this book could be considered energizing, so don't feel that you are limited to this section if you want to increase your energy. I created this section to draw your attention to the fact that fresh, raw juices can greatly improve your energy. They will all help you increase the nutrients and biophotons that energize your body.

The Morning Energizer

    4 carrots, scrubbed well, green tops removed, ends trimmed
    1 handful parsley
    1 lemon, peeled if not organic
    1 apple (green has less sugar)
    2-inch-chunk fresh ginger root, peeled

Cut produce to fit your juicer's feed tube. Juice all ingredients and stir. Pour into a glass and drink as soon as possible. Serves 1.

Energize-Your-Day Cocktail

    1 apple (green is lower in sugar)
    2 dark green leaves (chard, collard, or kale)
    1 stalk celery with leaves
    1 lemon, peeled if not organic
    ½ cucumber, peeled if not organic
    ½- to 1-inch-chunk fresh ginger root, peeled

Cut the apple into sections that fit your juicer's feed tube. Roll the green leaves and push through the feed tube with the apple, celery, lemon, cucumber, and ginger. Stir the juice and pour into a glass. Drink as soon as possible. Serves 1.

Happy-Mood Morning

Fennel juice has been used as a traditional tonic to help the body release endorphins, the "feel good" peptides, from the brain into the bloodstream. Endorphins help to diminish anxiety and fear and generate a mood of euphoria.

    ½ apple (green is lower in sugar)
    4-5 carrots, well scrubbed, green tops removed, ends trimmed
    3 fennel stalks with leaves and flowers
    ½ cucumber, peeled if not organic
    1 handful spinach
    1-inch-chunk ginger root

Cut produce to fit your juicer's feed tube. Juice apple first and follow with other ingredients. Stir and pour into a glass; drink as soon as possible. Serves 1–2.

Vitamin C–Rich Combinations

Vitamin C is important for a healthy immune system, detoxification, healthy adrenal glands, eyes, collagen, bone structure, cartilage, muscle, veins, capillaries, teeth, and gums. The richest sources of vitamin C include chili peppers, kale, parsley, collard greens, turnip greens, broccoli, mustard greens, watercress, spinach, lemon, and Swiss chard.

Carrot and Spice

2-3 carrots, scrubbed well, tops removed, ends trimmed
1 handful spinach
1 cucumber, peeled if not organic
½ lemon, peeled if not organic
½ apple (green has less sugar)
1-inch-chunk ginger root
¼ tsp. cinnamon
⅛ tsp. cayenne pepper

Cut produce to fit your juicer's feed tube. Juice all ingredients except spices. Pour juice into a glass, add spices, stir, and drink as soon as possible. Serves 2.

Raging Beet-Jalapeño

1 beet with tops
2 collard or Swiss chard leaves
1 cucumber, peeled if not organic
1 lemon, peeled if not organic
1-inch-chunk ginger root
½ small jalapeño, seeds removed

Cut produce to fit your juicer's feed tube. Juice the beet with its tops. Roll collard or chard leaves and follow with ½ cucumber. Add other ingredients and follow with the remaining cucumber. Pour juice into a glass, stir, and drink as soon as possible. Serves 1.

Peppy Parsley

1 cucumber, peeled if not organic
1 carrot, scrubbed well, green tops removed, ends trimmed
1 stalk celery with leaves
1 handful parsley
1 kale leaf
1 lemon, peeled if not organic

Cut produce to fit your juicer's feed tube. Juice the cucumber, carrot, and celery. Bunch up parsley and roll in kale leaf, add to juicer and push through. Then add lemon and juice. Stir and pour into a glass. Drink as soon as possible. Serves 1.

Detoxification Juices

Just as with the energizing recipes, all the juice recipes are detoxifying. But some have more specific action, which are included here. If you're embarking on a cleanse program, you can choose any of the recipes as part of your plan. For specific cleansing action, choose some of the recipes in this section.

Liver-Cleansing Cocktail

Beets have long been used to cleanse and support the liver. Be aware, however, that they are higher in sugar than most vegetables, as are carrots. You may need to use less beets and carrots if you have a sugar metabolism challenge and add more greens to the recipe to dilute the sugar.

> 3 carrots, scrubbed well, tops removed, ends trimmed
> 1 cucumber, peeled if not organic
> 1 beet with stem and leaves, scrubbed well
> 2 stalks celery
> 1 handful parsley
> 1- to 2-inch-chunk ginger root, scrubbed or peeled
> 1 lemon, peeled if not organic

Cut produce to fit your juicer's feed tube. Juice all ingredients and stir. Pour into a glass and drink as soon as possible. Serves 1-2.

Liver-Gallbladder Rejuvenator

Bitter herbs and foods such as dandelion leaves and citrus peel will stimulate and cleanse the liver.

> 3-4 carrots, scrubbed well, green tops removed, ends trimmed
> 1 cucumber, peeled if not organic
> 1 handful dandelion greens
> 1 lemon, with peel (choose only organic)
> ½ beet with leaves and stems, scrubbed well
> ½ green apple
> 1-inch-chunk ginger

Cut produce to fit your juicer's feed tube. Juice all ingredients and stir. Pour into a glass and drink as soon as possible. Serves 1-2.

Liver Life Tonic

Dandelion juice is a traditional remedy for cleansing the liver.

1 handful dandelion greens
3–4 carrots, scrubbed well, tops removed, ends trimmed
1 cucumber, peeled if not organic
1 lemon, peeled if not organic

Cut produce to fit your juicer's feed tube. Bunch up dandelion greens. Tuck the greens in feed tube and push through with a carrot. Juice the remaining ingredients. Stir the juice, pour into a glass, and drink as soon as possible. Serves 1.

Natural Diuretic Tonic

Cucumber, asparagus, and lemon are all natural diuretics. Getting rid of old stored-up water is a great boost to your cleansing program.

1 medium vine-ripened tomato
1 cucumber, peeled if not organic
8 asparagus stems
1 lemon or lime, peeled if not organic
Dash hot sauce

Cut produce to fit your juicer's feed tube. Juice all ingredients except hot sauce. Pour into a glass, stir in hot sauce, and drink as soon as possible. Serves 1.

Happy Colon Tonic

1 green apple or pear
1 cucumber, peeled if not organic
1 lemon, peeled if not organic
1 handful spinach
1 handful parsley

Cut produce to fit your juicer's feed tube. Juice all ingredients and stir. Pour into a glass and drink as soon as possible. Serves 1–2.

Juice Recipes for Diabetics and Prediabetics

I've often heard people say they can't juice because they have diabetes. You can juice vegetables if you have sugar metabolism problems, but you should choose low-sugar veggies and only low-sugar fruits such as lemons, limes, and cranberries. Carrots and beets would be too high in sugar. You could add one or two carrots to a juice recipe or a very small beet or part of a beet, but they should be diluted with cucumber juice and dark leafy greens. You may use cranberries, lemons, and limes, but other fruits are higher in sugar and should be avoided. Berries are low in sugar, especially blueberries, and can be added to juice recipes. Green apples are lower in sugar than yellow or red apples. But I don't recommend that you use even green apples unless you have your blood sugar under control. Keep your juices very low in sugar.

I've worked with people who have reversed their diabetes by juicing low-sugar vegetables and eating many more living foods, along with a low-glycemic, high-fiber diet.

Sprinkle cinnamon in your juice

Researchers have suggested that people with diabetes may see improvements by adding ¼ to 1 teaspoon of cinnamon to their food. A twelve-week London study involved fifty-eight type 2 diabetics. After twelve weeks on 2 grams (about ½ teaspoon) of cinnamon per day, study subjects had significantly lowered blood sugar levels, as well as significantly reduced blood pressures.[1]

Broccoli Surprise

Broccoli could help reverse the damage that diabetes inflicts on blood vessels. The key is likely a compound in the vegetable called sulforaphane. It encourages production of enzymes that protect the blood vessels and reduce the number of molecules that cause cell damage, known as reactive oxygen species (ROS), by up to 73 percent.

- 2–3 carrots, scrubbed well, tops removed, ends trimmed
- 2–3 broccoli florets or 1 broccoli stem
- 2 celery stalks, with leaves as desired
- ½ cucumber, scrubbed well
- ½ lemon, peeled if not organic

Cut produce to fit your juicer's feed tube. Juice all ingredients and stir. Pour into a glass and drink as soon as possible. Serves 1.

NOTE: Save all broccoli stems and juice them; you can add them to most recipes and reap the rewards. This is good economy and adds great nutrition.

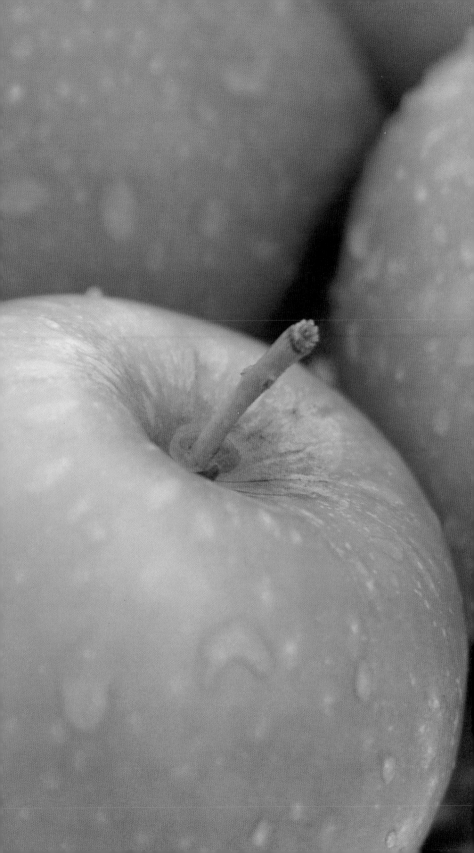

Magnesium-Rich Cocktail

A new study out of the University of North Carolina at Chapel Hill points to a connection between magnesium in the diet and lowered risk of diabetes.[2]

- 4-5 beet tops
- 2 Swiss chard leaves
- 2 collard leaves
- 1 cucumber, peeled if not organic
- ½ cup blueberries, thawed if frozen
- ½ lemon, peeled if not organic

Cut produce to fit your juicer's feed tube. Turn off the machine when adding the blueberries. Put the plunger in place, then turn the machine on and juice, followed by the lemon. Stir. Pour into a glass and drink as soon as possible. Serves 2.

Healing Juices

Adrenal Booster Cocktail

Hot peppers and parsley are rich in vitamin C; celery is a great source of natural sodium. Both are very beneficial for the adrenal glands.

- 4 carrots, scrubbed well, green tops removed, ends trimmed
- 2 tomatoes
- 2 stalks celery
- 1 handful parsley
- Dash of hot sauce
- Dash of celery salt

Cut produce to fit your juicer's feed tube. Juice all ingredients and stir. Pour into a glass and drink as soon as possible. Serves 2.

Allergy Relief

Parsley is a traditional remedy for allergic reactions. You need to juice a bunch as soon as possible after a reaction occurs. It can help open airways when sipped.

- 1 bunch parsley
- 2 celery stalks
- 1-2 carrots, scrubbed well, tops removed, ends trimmed
- 1 lemon, peeled if not organic
- ½ cucumber, peeled if not organic

Cut produce to fit your juicer's feed tube. Juice all ingredients and stir. Pour into a glass and drink as soon as possible. Serves 1.

Healthy Bones Cocktail

Kale and parsley are loaded with calcium, but that's not all. They also have magnesium, boron, and vitamin K—all are important for bone health.

1 cucumber, peeled if not organic
1 large kale leaf
1 chard leaf
1 handful parsley
1 celery stalk
1 lemon, peeled if not organic
1-inch-chunk ginger root, scrubbed or peeled if old

Cut produce to fit your juicer's feed tube. Juice all ingredients and stir. Pour into a glass and drink as soon as possible. Serves 1.

Cancer Fighter

A team in the UK found that a compound in carrots called falcarinol reduced cancer in rats.[3] Allicin, a compound in garlic, has also been found to fight cancer.[4]

1-2 carrots, scrubbed well, green tops removed, ends trimmed
1-2 kale leaves
½ cucumber, peeled if not organic
1 garlic clove with peel
1 handful watercress or parsley, rinsed
1 lemon, peeled if not organic

Cut produce to fit your juicer's feed tube. Juice carrots. Roll kale leaves and push through with cucumber; add garlic, watercress or parsley, and push through with lemon. Stir and drink as soon as possible. Serves 1.

Triple C Ulcer Mender

Scientific research has proven that cabbage juice is an effective treatment for stomach ulcers.[5] By itself it does not taste good, but with about equal parts of carrot and celery, it has a slightly nutty taste. (Avoid citrus if you have an ulcer; they can aggravate symptoms.)

¼ small head green cabbage
3 carrots, scrubbed well, tops removed, ends trimmed
4 celery stalks, with leaves if desired

Cut produce to fit your juicer's feed tube. Juice all ingredients and stir. You will need to drink this right away as cabbage juice does not store well. Serves 1.

Cabbage Patch (Ulcer Healer)

Sulforaphane is a compound in cabbage, broccoli, cauliflower, and kale, which has been reported to inhibit antibiotic-resistant strains of *Helicobacter pylori* (which cause ulcers). Broccoli sprouts contain from thirty to fifty times the concentration of this chemical as in the mature plants. This effect was identified by scientists at the Johns Hopkins University School of Medicine in Baltimore while investigating sulforaphane for its protective effect against cancer.[6]

3 stalks celery with leaves
3 carrots, scrubbed well, tops removed, ends trimmed
1 cucumber, peeled if not organic
1 lemon, peeled if not organic
¼ green cabbage (spring or summer cabbage is best)
Handful broccoli sprouts (optional)

Cut produce to fit your juicer's feed tube. Juice all ingredients and stir. Pour into a glass and drink as soon as possible. Serves 1.

The Pink Onion
(Stomach Cancer and Ulcer Fighter)

The odorous sulfur compounds found in onions help fight the *H. pylori* bacteria, which is linked with ulcers and stomach cancer.

3 carrots, scrubbed well, tops removed, ends trimmed
2 stalks celery
1 small beet with tops
1 cucumber, peeled if not organic
½ sweet onion
½ pear

Cut produce to fit your juicer's feed tube. Juice all ingredients and stir. Pour into a glass and drink as soon as possible. Serves 2.

Flu Mender

Garlic is a natural antibiotic and antibacterial with reports going back through history. It can be quite effective as a broad-spectrum antibiotic. One significant advantage of garlic is that the bacteria do not seem to build up a resistance to it as they do to many modern antibiotics. Old or cooked garlic loses its effectiveness; only raw, crushed garlic works.

1 cucumber, peeled if not organic
1–2 carrots, scrubbed well, tops removed, ends trimmed
1–2 cloves garlic
1 lemon, peeled if not organic

Cut produce to fit your juicer's feed tube. Juice all ingredients and stir. Pour into a glass and drink as soon as possible. Serves 1.

Folic Acid–Rich Cocktail (for a Healthy Baby)

Planning on getting pregnant? Folic acid is important to prevent birth defects. Parsnips are rich in folic acid. This B vitamin also plays a role in reducing heart disease and may help prevent dementia and osteoporosis.

    2-3 carrots, scrubbed well, tops removed, ends trimmed
    1 cucumber, peeled if not organic
    1 small parsnip
    1 lemon, peeled if not organic

Cut produce to fit your juicer's feed tube. Juice all ingredients and stir. Pour into a glass and drink as soon as possible. Serves 1.

Cran-Apple Cocktail (Kidney-Bladder Helper)

Cranberries have been shown to fight urinary tract infections, binding to bacteria so it cannot latch on to the bladder wall. It helps to cleanse the kidneys and is a natural diuretic.

    2 organic green apples
    ¼ to ½ cup fresh or frozen (thawed) cranberries
    ½ cucumber, peeled if not organic
    ½ lemon, peeled if not organic
    1-inch-chunk ginger root
    ¼ cup purified water (optional)

Cut produce to fit your juicer's feed tube. Juice 1 apple first. Turn off the machine, add the cranberries, and put the plunger in; then turn the machine on and juice. Follow with the lemon, ginger, and second apple. Add water as needed. Stir and pour into a glass; drink as soon as possible. Serves 1-2.

Gallstone Solvent Cocktail

There is evidence that magnesium helps prevent and dissolve gallstones. One natural way to alleviate a gallbladder attack is to drink a glass of water at the start of the attack. Then follow by taking magnesium followed by bitter liquid such as Swedish bitters and/or bitter green juice an hour later. Bitter flavors stimulate bile flow.

    1 apple (green has less sugar)
    Several bitter green leaves such as dandelion, arugula, rapini,
      or mustard
    3-4 dark leafy greens (rich in magnesium) such as chard or
      collard greens
    1 cucumber, peeled if not organic
    1 lemon, peeled if not organic
    1 carrot, scrubbed well, green tops removed, ends trimmed

Cut produce to fit your juicer's feed tube. Juice the apple. Roll the green leaves and push through feed tube followed by remaining ingredients. Juice ingredients and stir. Pour into a glass and drink as soon as possible. Serves 1.

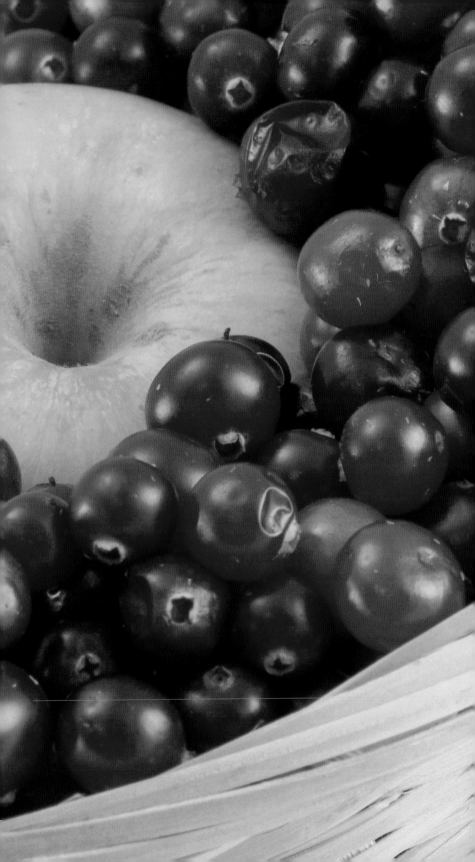

Gout Fighter

Cherries help reduce uric acid in the bloodstream and help prevent inflammation caused by gout. Parsley, a natural diuretic, helps flush away uric acid.

1 green apple,
½ pound cherries, pits removed (if frozen, thaw first)
2 stalks celery with leaves, as desired
1 handful parsley
1 lemon, peeled if not organic

Cut produce to fit your juicer's feed tube. Juice all ingredients and stir. Pour into a glass and drink as soon as possible. Serves 1.

Garlic Wonder Flu and Cold Mender

1 handful parsley
1 dark green lettuce leaf such as green leaf or romaine
½ cucumber, peeled if not organic
1 garlic clove
3 carrots, scrubbed well, green tops removed, ends trimmed
2 stalks celery with leaves, as desired
1 lemon, peeled if not organic

Cut produce to fit your juicer's feed tube. Roll parsley in lettuce leaf. Juice cucumber, then parsley rolled in lettuce leaf. Add garlic and push through juicer with carrots, followed by celery and lemon. Stir and pour into a glass. Serves 1.

Lung Rejuvenator

Turnip juice has been used as a traditional remedy to strengthen lung tissue. Pear is also known to be good for the lungs.

1 handful watercress or parsley
1 small turnip, scrubbed well, tops removed, ends trimmed
1 pear
2 carrots, scrubbed well, tops removed, ends trimmed
1 garlic clove
½ lemon, peeled if not organic

Bunch up watercress or parsley. Cut produce to fit your juicer's feed tube. Tuck the watercress or parsley in feed tube and push through with the turnip. Juice remaining ingredients, finishing with a carrot. Stir the juice, pour into a glass, and drink as soon as possible. Serves 1.

Healthy Sinus Solution

Radish juice is a traditional remedy to open up the sinuses and support mucous membranes. The best sinus healer is a liver cleanse.

2 tomatoes
6 radishes
1 lime, peeled if not organic
½ cucumber, peeled if not organic

Cut produce to fit your juicer's feed tube. Juice all ingredients and stir. Pour into a glass and drink as soon as possible. Serves 1.

Memory Tonic

The most powerful vegetables for improving memory include the cruciferous vegetables (cauliflower, broccoli, brussels sprouts, cabbage, kale); green leafy vegetables; purple fruits and vegetables (rich in anthocyanins) such as beets, blueberries, and purple cabbage; and quercetin-rich red fruits and vegetables such as red apples, tomatoes, and red onions.

    3 dark green leafy vegetables such as chard, collards, kale
    3 cauliflower florets or cauliflower base (that you might
        otherwise toss)
    1 cucumber, peeled if not organic
    1 beet with green leaves
    1 lemon, peeled if not organic
    1 red apple

Cut produce to fit your juicer's feed tube. Roll the green leaves and push through the hopper with the remaining ingredients. Juice all ingredients and stir. Pour into a glass and drink as soon as possible. Serves 1–2.

Mood Mender

Fennel juice has been used as a traditional tonic to help the body release endorphins, the "feel good" peptides from the brain into the bloodstream. Endorphins help to diminish anxiety and fear and generate a mood of euphoria.

    3 fennel stalks with leaves
    3 carrots, scrubbed well, tops removed, ends trimmed
    2 stalks celery with leaves, as desired
    ½ pear
    1-inch-chunk ginger root, peeled

Cut produce to fit your juicer's feed tube. Juice all ingredients and stir. Pour into a glass and drink as soon as possible. Serves 1–2.

Pancreas Helper

Brussels sprouts and string bean juice have been used as traditional remedies to help strengthen and support the pancreas. Drink before a meal. (If this drink is too strong, dilute with a little water.)

    1 large tomato
    2 romaine lettuce leaves
    8 string beans
    2 brussels sprouts
    1 lemon, peeled if not organic

Cut produce to fit your juicer's feed tube. Juice all ingredients and stir. Pour into a glass and drink as soon as possible. Serves 1–2.

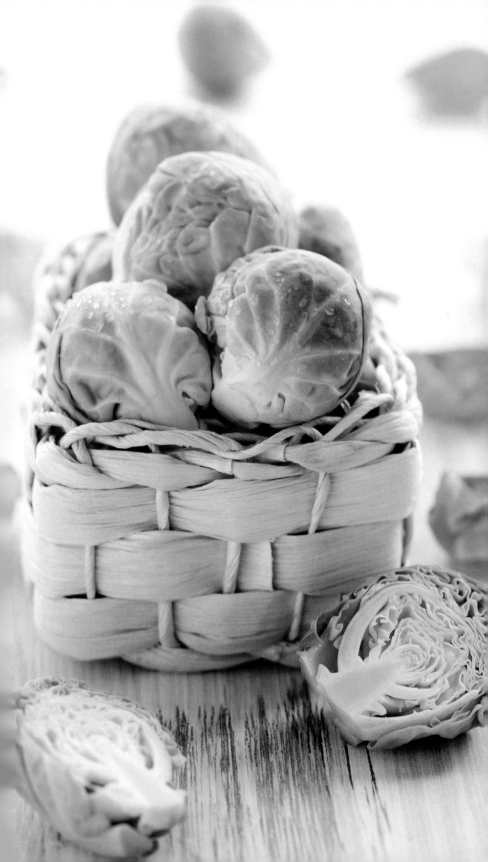

Sweet Sleep Cocktail

Lettuce and celery help the body relax and help you sleep more deeply.

> 5 medium carrots, scrubbed well, green tops removed, ends trimmed
> 2 stalks celery
> 2 romaine lettuce leaves
> 1 kale leaf
> 1 lemon, peeled if not organic
> ½ green apple, optional

Cut produce to fit your juicer's feed tube. Juice all ingredients and stir. Pour into a glass and drink as soon as possible. Serves 1.

Sweet Regularity With a Twist

> 1 pear
> 1 apple
> 1 cucumber, peeled if not organic
> ½ lemon, peeled if not organic

Cut produce to fit your juicer's feed tube. Juice all ingredients and stir. Pour into a glass and drink as soon as possible. Serves 1-2.

The Pancreas Revitalizer

String beans are a traditional remedy for the pancreas. They are especially good for people with diabetes.

> 2 tomatoes
> 1 cucumber, peeled if not organic
> 6–8 string beans
> 1 lemon or lime, peeled if not organic
> Dash of hot sauce

Cut produce to fit your juicer's feed tube. Juice all ingredients and stir. Pour into a glass and drink as soon as possible. Serves 1.

Thyroid Tonic

Radishes are a traditional tonic for the thyroid gland.

> 5 carrots, scrubbed well, green tops removed, ends trimmed
> 5–6 radishes
> 1 lemon, peeled if not organic
> ½ cucumber, peeled if not organic

Cut produce to fit your juicer's feed tube. Juice all ingredients and stir. Pour into a glass and drink as soon as possible. Serves 1.

Smoothies

Green Berry Blast

    1 cucumber, peeled if not organic
    ½ apple
    1 cup berries (blueberries, raspberries, or blackberries) fresh or
        frozen
    3-4 dark green leaves (collards, Swiss chard, or kale)
    1-inch-chunk ginger root
    ½ lemon, peeled if not organic (Meyers lemons are sweeter)
    1 avocado

Cut the cucumber and apple in chunks. Place the cucumber, apple, and berries in a blender and process until smooth. Chop the greens and ginger and add to the blender along with the juice of half a lemon; process until smooth. Add the avocado and process until well blended. Serves 2.

Green Coconut Delight
(Yeast-Fat Buster Smoothie)

Coconut oil is an ally in breaking the yeast-fat cycle. One study showed that it destroyed *Candida albicans* on contact.[7] Its fatty acids split open the protective outer coating of yeast cells.

    1 cucumber cut in chunks, peeled if not organic
    1 cup raw spinach, kale, or chard, chopped
    1 avocado, peeled, seeded, and cut in quarters
    ½ cup coconut milk
    1 Tbsp. virgin coconut oil
    Juice of 1 lime or lemon

Combine all ingredients in a blender and process until creamy. Serves 2.

Kale-Pear Smoothie

Kale is packed with calcium in a form that is assimilated by the body far better than the calcium in dairy products—and that's a great bonus for your bones!

    1 cucumber, peeled if not organic
    1 cup kale
    2 pears (Asian or Bartlett)
    1 avocado
    6 ice cubes

Chop cucumber, kale, and pears and place in the blender; process until smooth. Add the avocado and ice and blend until creamy. Serves 2.

Healthy Green Smoothie

 1 cucumber, peeled if not organic
 2 stalks celery
 1 handful of kale, parsley, or spinach
 1 green apple
 ½ lemon, peeled if not organic
 6 ice cubes

Chop the cucumber, celery, greens, and apple. Place in blender with lemon and ice; process until creamy. Serves 2.

Sprouted Almond-Vanilla Smoothie

 1 cup raw almonds, soaked overnight
 1 cup unsweetened almond milk
 1 cup berries (blueberries, strawberries, or blackberries), fresh or
    frozen
 ½ tsp. pure vanilla extract
 6 ice cubes

Soak almonds in water overnight so that they will sprout. (Sprouting allows the almond to partially germinate, which removes the enzyme inhibitors and increases nutrient value.) Blend together almonds, almond milk, berries, vanilla, and ice. Pour into glasses and serve as soon as possible. Serves 2.

Cranberry-Pear Fat Buster Smoothie

 2 pears, Bartlett or Asian
 ½ cucumber, peeled if not organic
 ¼ lemon, peeled if not organic
 2 Tbsp. cranberries, fresh or frozen
 ½- to 1-inch-chunk ginger root
 6 ice cubes (optional)

Chop up pears and cucumber and blend until smooth. Add lemon, cranberries, ginger, and ice as desired; blend until creamy. Serves 1.

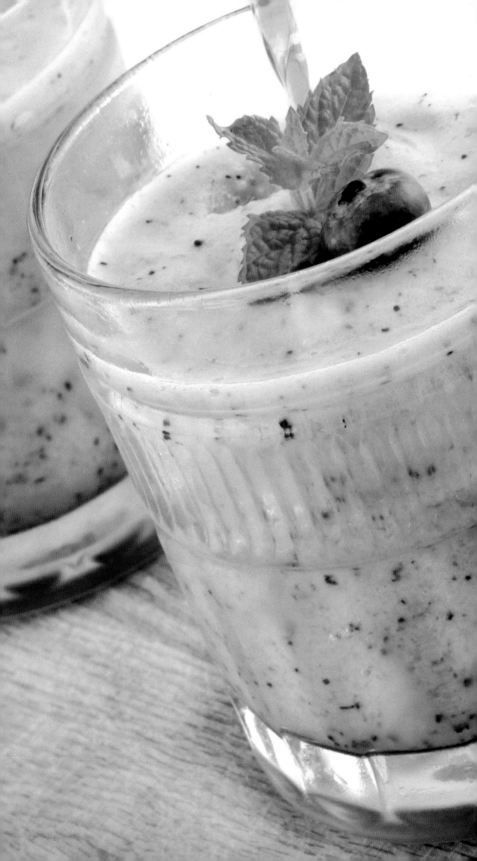

Nutty Delight

Parsley is rich in vitamin C, bioflavonoids, beta-carotene, iron, calcium, magnesium, potassium, zinc, and vanadium. Couple that with bromelain from the pineapple juice and protein and essential fatty acids from the nuts, and you have a super meal-in-a-glass.

    10 raw almonds
    1 Tbsp. sunflower seeds
    1 Tbsp. sesame seeds
    1 Tbsp. flaxseeds
    1 Tbsp. chia seeds (optional)
    1 cup pineapple juice (juice half a pineapple)
    1 cup chopped parsley
    ½ cup milk of choice
    ½ tsp. pure vanilla extract
    1 Tbsp. protein powder (optional)
    6 ice cubes

Place the nuts, seeds, and pineapple juice in a bowl; cover and soak overnight. (See Health Tip below.) Place this nut and seed mixture with the juice in a blender and add the parsley, milk, vanilla, protein powder (as desired), and ice cubes. Blend on high speed until smooth. This drink will be a bit chewy because of the nuts and seeds. Serves 2.

HEALTH TIP: To kill molds, soak nuts and seeds for one hour to overnight in water or juice to which you add ½ teaspoon ascorbic acid (vitamin C powder). In this case you will add it to the pineapple juice.

Dr. Nina's Sweet Dandelion Smoothie

    1 pear, Bartlett or Asian
    1 apple (green has less sugar)
    1 large handful dandelion greens
    1 cup coconut milk
    Juice of ½ lemon
    ¼ cup flaxseeds
    6 ice cubes (optional)

Place all ingredients in a blender and process until a creamy shake. Serves 2.

Cold Soups

Borscht in the Raw

    6 tomatoes
    2 beets
    3 carrots
    3 stalks of celery
    2 Tbsp. lemon juice
    3 oranges, peeled, or 1 peach
    1 Tbsp. honey or 4 dates, pitted
    ½ cup extra-virgin olive oil

½ cup chopped parsley
1–2 cups water, as needed
1 cup raw walnuts
½ head cabbage and 1 beet, grated and set aside for later

Juice the tomatoes, beets, carrots, and celery together. In a blender, combine the juice plus lemon juice, peeled oranges or peach, sweetener, olive oil, parsley, and water, if needed. Pulse in the walnuts, leaving a nutty consistency. Pour in individual serving dishes and add the grated cabbage and beets into each one. Serves 2.

Red Bell Pepper Soup

¼ cup water
Juice of ½ lemon
1 small cucumber, peeled if not organic
1 green onion, chopped
⅓ cup parsley, chopped
⅓ cup cilantro, chopped
1 clove garlic
2 Tbsp. extra-virgin olive oil
1 pinch Celtic sea salt
1 large red bell pepper

Blend all ingredients together in a blender until smooth. Serves 2.

Icy Spicy Gazpacho

Chili peppers actually induce the brain to secrete endorphins, those brain chemicals that are credited with the "runner's high." Endorphins block pain sensations and induce a kind of euphoria. When you're feeling great, you're less likely to go on a food binge.

2 tomatoes, cut in chunks
1 cup fresh carrot juice (about 5–7 carrots)
1 lemon, juiced, peeled if putting it through a juice machine
½ bunch cilantro, rinsed and chopped
¼ tsp. Celtic sea salt
¼ tsp. ground cumin
¼ small jalapeño, chopped (more if you like it hot)

Place the tomato chunks in a freezer bag and freeze until solid. Pour the carrot and lemon juices into a blender and add the frozen tomato chunks, cilantro, salt, cumin, and jalapeño. Blend on high speed until smooth, but slushy; serve immediately. Serves 2.

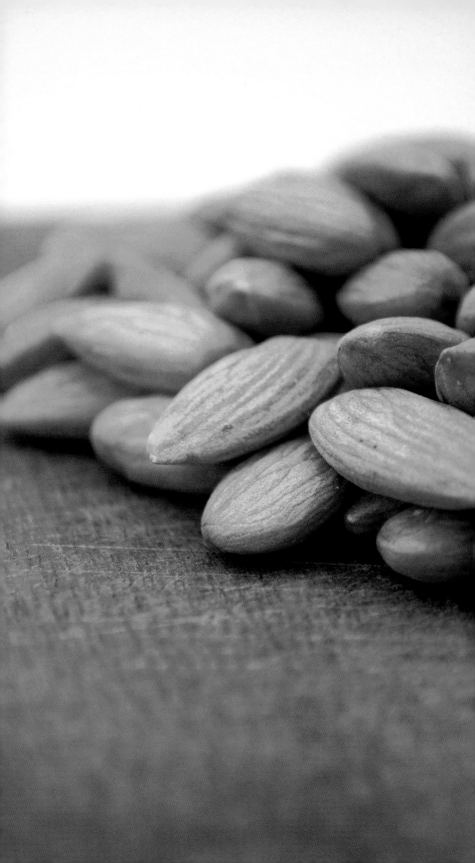

Breakfasts

Buckwheat Granola

½ cup fresh orange juice
¼ cup honey or pure maple syrup, adjust to taste
2 tsp. vanilla
1 tsp. cinnamon
1 apple, chopped (optional)
1 cup dried coconut
1 cup chopped raw almonds
1 cup chopped raw walnuts
1 cup raw sunflower seeds
1 cup raw sesame seeds
1 cup wheat germ
2 cups dehydrated buckwheat groats (see Note)
1 vanilla bean (optional)

Mix orange juice, honey, vanilla, cinnamon, and apple (if using) in blender. Set aside. In a bowl, place coconut, almonds, walnuts, sunflower seeds, sesame seeds, wheat germ, and dehydrated buckwheat groats. Pour blended ingredients over entire mixture. Toss well to coat all the dry ingredients. Scoop in clumps onto P-Flexx sheets. Dehydrate at 105 degrees for about 8 hours or until tops are crunchy. Turn over and dehydrate until tops are crunchy. Makes 6 cups.

NOTE: In a large jar or bowl, soak raw buckwheat groats (about 2 cups) overnight. Drain and rinse in colander. Cover colander with lightweight cotton dishtowel; continue to rinse several times a day for the next day. Place groats on P-Flexx sheet and dehydrate overnight at 105 degrees. Store with a vanilla bean in a jar covered with lid.

Apple Muesli

Oats are a good source of B vitamins, vitamin E, manganese, zinc, selenium, nickel, molybdenum, and vanadium. Oats contain gluten (substitute buckwheat groats, if gluten sensitive) and phytates, a binding agent that can cause some mineral loss if consumed frequently. Soaking grains overnight, as recommended here, breaks down some of the phytic acid in the bran.

½ cup raisins
¼ cup rolled oats
2 Tbsp. sunflower seeds
2 Tbsp. flaxseeds
2 Tbsp. bee pollen
½ tsp. ascorbic acid (vitamin C powder)
½ cup milk of choice
½ cup chopped apple
½ tsp. cinnamon extract or ground cinnamon

Place raisins, oats, sunflower seeds, flaxseeds, bee pollen, and ascorbic acid in a bowl and cover with milk. Cover the bowl and let soak overnight in the refrigerator. Add chopped apple and cinnamon before serving. Makes about 1½ cups.

Lemon Muesli

Flaxseeds are rich in omega-3 fatty acids and are one of the richest sources of lignans. To release these heart-healthy nutrients from the hard coating of the flaxseed, it must be ground in a blender or nut grinder. Otherwise, the flaxseed will pass right through your body without much benefit.

- ¼ cup rolled oats
- ¼ cup raisins
- 2 Tbsp. almonds
- 2 Tbsp. flaxseeds
- ½ tsp. ascorbic acid (vitamin C powder)
- ½ cup milk of choice
- 1 Tbsp. fresh lemon juice
- 1 tsp. freshly grated lemon peel, preferably organic

Place the oats, raisins, almonds, flaxseed, and vitamin C in a bowl; pour the milk over them. Cover the bowl and refrigerate overnight. Add the lemon juice and zest before serving and stir. Makes about 1 cup.

Sprouted Buckwheat Groats

Put 1 cup (or as much as you want) of raw buckwheat groat seeds into a bowl or your sprouter. Add 2-3 times as much cool, purified water. Swish seeds around to assure even water contact for all. Allow seeds to soak for 6-8 hours. Drain off the soak water. Rinse thoroughly with cool water. Groats create very starchy water; it's very thick! They won't sprout well unless rinsed well, so rinse until the water runs clear. Drain thoroughly. You can add to your sprouter at this time or simply put the sprouts in a colander and cover with a tea towel. Set out of direct sunlight at room temperature (70 degrees is optimal). Rinse and drain again in 4-8 hours. Yields approximately 1½ cups of sprouts.

For your morning cereal, sprouted buckwheat is great served with rice, oat, or almond milk and a sprinkle of ground almonds and cinnamon. You can also dehydrate sprouted groats for a crunchy cereal.

Salads

Walnut Zucchini Greens

- 1 head of broccoli, lightly blanch broccoli florets under hot tap
  water until they turn bright green
- 2 small zucchini, finely shredded in food processor
- 1 red pepper, finely chopped
- 2 cups torn romaine or green leaf lettuce
- ½ cup walnuts, chopped
- Ginger-Lime Dressing (page 199)

Mix first three ingredients in bowl. Then place veggies on the bed of greens. Sprinkle walnuts over top. Drizzle dressing over salad. Serves 4.

Apple Fennel Salad With Lemon Zest

2 cups fennel, sliced julienne thin
2 cups apple, sliced julienne thin
2 Tbsp. fresh lemon juice
2 Tbsp. lemon zest
2 Tbsp. extra-virgin olive oil
2 Tbsp. fresh, minced thyme
1 sliver of jalapeño, minced
1 tsp. Celtic sea salt

Place the fennel and apple slices in a bowl; set aside. In a small bowl, whisk together lemon juice, zest, olive oil, thyme, jalapeño, and salt. Pour dressing over fennel-apple mixture and toss. Serves 4.

Winter Salad

1 large grapefruit
2 small fresh fennel bulbs, trimmed, halved vertically, sliced
    paper-thin (save discarded parts for juicing)
1 cup fresh parsley, chopped
Lemon-Ginger Dressing (page 199)

Peel grapefruit and cut off white part. Separate segments and slice into pieces. Combine grapefruit, fennel, and parsley. Add dressing to taste and toss. Serves 2.

Dr. Nina's Russian Cabbage Slaw

4 cups shredded cabbage
1 cup grated carrot
½ cup dandelion greens or watercress, chopped
4 cloves garlic, minced
Juice of ½ lemon
¼ cup extra-virgin olive oil

Place the cabbage, carrot, greens, and garlic in a bowl; set aside. In a small bowl, whisk together lemon juice and olive oil. Pour over the cabbage mixture and toss well. Serves 4.

Broccoli-Cauliflower Slaw

1 cup broccoli florets
1 cup cauliflower florets
½ red sweet onion, chopped
1 carrot, chopped
½ tsp. Celtic sea salt
Pinch of dill weed
½ cup Cashew Mayonnaise (page 200)

Put all ingredients except mayonnaise in the food processor and pulse until they are like "slaw." Stir in Cashew Mayonnaise. Serves 2.

Sprouted Quinoa Salad

Quinoa is a seed, not a grain, but it can substitute for any grain. It is high in protein, complete with all eight essential amino acids, and it's gluten free.

    2 cups sprouted quinoa
    2 avocados, diced
    2 tomatoes, diced
    1 clove garlic minced
    ½ cup chopped cilantro (optional)
    3 Tbsp. nutritional yeast
    1 tsp. cumin
    ½ tsp. Celtic sea salt
    Juice of 1 lime

Soak quinoa overnight and then sprout for 2 days. Put quinoa in a bowl with remaining ingredients. Toss and serve on a bed of greens or in raw burritos. Serves 4.

Ginger-Beet Salad

    4 cups grated beets
    1 Tbsp. grated ginger root
    ¼ cup extra-virgin olive oil
    ¼ cup fresh lemon juice

Finely grate beets in food processor. or with grater. In small bowl, combine beets, ginger, olive oil, and lemon juice. Toss and let the flavors blend for a few minutes before serving. Serves 4.

Dressings, Sauces, Dips, and Condiments

Sunflower Dill Sauce

    2 cups raw sunflower seeds, soaked for 8–12 hours
    ⅔ cup lemon juice or 1 cucumber, peeled
    ⅓ cup extra-virgin olive oil
    2 Tbsp. minced garlic
    1 tsp. Celtic sea salt
    6 Tbsp. fresh, chopped dill or 2 Tbsp. dried dill

In a high-speed blender, blend sunflower seeds, lemon juice or cucumber, olive oil, garlic, and salt until smooth. Pulse in the dill. More cucumber may be added for desired consistency if needed. Makes about 3–3¼ cups.

Lemon-Ginger Dressing

    2 lemons, juiced
    2-inch-chunk ginger root, grated
    ½ cup extra-virgin olive oil
    2 cloves garlic, peeled and crushed
    3 Tbsp. miso
    2 Tbsp. shoyu
    2–3 Tbsp. raw honey or pure maple syrup

Mix all ingredients in blender. If needed, add water to thin. Makes 1 cup.

Ginger-Lime Dressing

    ¼ cup fresh lime juice
    ¼ cup sesame oil
    ¼ cup purified water
    2 Tbsp. tamari
    2 Tbsp. fresh mint
    1 Tbsp. fresh cilantro
    1 tsp. ginger root
    1 thin slice red chili pepper or dash of cayenne pepper
    1 Tbsp. pure maple syrup
    1 tsp. Celtic sea salt

Combine all the ingredients in a blender and blend well. Makes about 1 cup.

Sesame Dressing

    ½ cup cold-pressed sesame oil
    1 Tbsp. grated ginger
    1 Tbsp. tamari or shoyu
    4 garlic cloves, minced
    ¼ cup rice vinegar
    1 Tbsp. pure maple syrup
    1 tsp. mustard
    Dash cayenne
    ¼–½ cup purified water

Place all ingredients in a blender and process until well combined. Makes about 1 cup.

Creamy Green Dressing

1 tsp. honey or pure maple syrup
2 Tbsp. fresh lemon juice
⅓ cup purified water
1 cup parsley, chopped
2 cloves garlic, chopped
⅓ cup cashews (not soaked)
1 tsp. Celtic sea salt
Juice of ½ small orange

Place all ingredients in a blender and process until well combined. Makes about 1 cup.

Cashew Mayonnaise

1 cup raw cashews, soaked overnight
Juice of 1 lemon
1 tsp. Celtic sea salt
½ tsp. onion powder
½ tsp. dill weed
Water as needed

Put all ingredients in blender with water just barely covering the cashews. Blend until smooth. Taste and adjust seasoning if necessary. Makes about 1½ cups.

Healthy Raw Ketchup

Studies involving the tomato have cropped up all over the world. It's rich in lycopene, an antioxidant that helps fight against cancer cell formation as well as other kinds of health complications and diseases.

1 cup chopped tomato
1 cup sun-dried tomatoes, soaked for 30 minutes, drained, and chopped
1 Tbsp. fresh garlic, minced
10 fresh basil leaves
3 dates, pitted
¼ cup extra-virgin olive oil
1 Tbsp. shoyu or 1 tsp. Celtic sea salt
1–2 Tbsp. Bragg's raw, unfiltered apple cider vinegar

Blend all ingredients together until it forms a paste. Makes about 2½ cups.

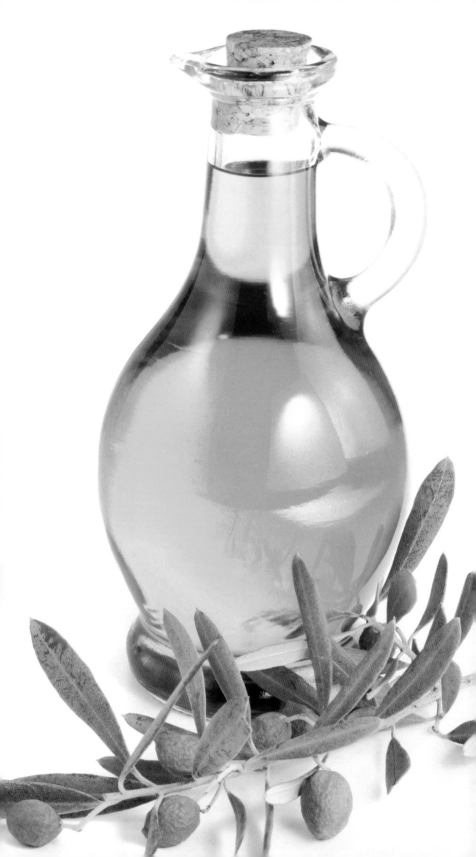

Raw Pesto Sauce

½–¾ cup organic raw pine nuts
¼ cup fresh organic fresh basil, de-stemmed
2 Tbsp. extra-virgin olive oil
1–2 Tbsp. fresh lemon juice
1–2 garlic cloves
1 tsp. Celtic sea salt
¼ cup purified water, reserved

Add all the ingredients to a food processor or blender. Pulse the mixture in food processor or blender, adding 1 tablespoon of water at a time to help facilitate blending and in order to reach the desired consistency for the sauce. Makes about 1¼ cups.

Nutty Cheese Sauce

1 cup macadamia nuts and 1 cup raw pine nuts, soaked or
   2 cups cashews, soaked (cashews are a bit sweeter and
   usually less expensive)
½ cup fresh lemon juice
1½ tsp. Celtic sea salt
1 Tbsp. garlic, chopped
½ tsp. ground peppercorns (optional)
Purified water as needed (usually between ¼ and ½ cup)

Soak nuts first for several hours. Blend all ingredients until very creamy. Blend for about 3 to 4 minutes for the creamiest sauce. Add water as needed. This sauce will keep 3 days in the refrigerator in a covered container. Makes 1½ cups.

Marinara Sauce

1 cup sun-dried tomatoes
1½ cups blended tomatoes
2 Tbsp. chopped onion
2 garlic cloves, peeled
2 Tbsp. extra-virgin olive oil
½ cup fresh lemon juice
Celtic sea salt, to taste

Combine all the ingredients in a blender and process until desired consistency is reached. Makes about 3 cups.

Raw Almond Mayo

2 cups raw almonds, soaked overnight
4 Tbsp. maple syrup or agave nectar
½ cup water
Juice of 2 lemons
1 tsp. onion or garlic powder
1 tsp. Celtic sea salt
¼ cup fresh basil
¼ cup extra-virgin olive oil (optional)

In a food processor, thoroughly blend almonds with maple syrup, water, and lemon juice. Add remaining ingredients. If mixture needs to be thickened, slowly add oil while processing. Makes about 3½ cups.

Mexican Almond Dip

1 cup almonds, soaked
½–1 tsp. Celtic sea salt
½ small sweet onion
½ clove elephant garlic with the center removed
¼ tsp. chili powder
¼–½ tsp. cumin
Water, as needed for desired consistency

Soak the almonds, covered, a day ahead, changing the water once. Mix all ingredients in a food processor. Serve on romaine leaves with Chef Avi Dalene's Green Tortillas (page 211) or Awesome Corn Crackers (page 207). Makes about 1¼ cups.

Almond Filling

2 cups almonds, soaked 7–8 hours, rinsed well
1 carrot, with cut ends and peeled, chopped (if using food processor)
2 stalks celery, cut ends, finely minced
1 medium red pepper, finely minced, with seeds and ribs removed
1 small onion, finely minced

Using a juicer with a blank blade such as the Champion or the Omega, or a food processor, homogenize the almonds and carrot, catching them in a large bowl. Or place the soaked almonds and carrot in a food processor and blend until homogenized. To this mixture add celery, red pepper, and onion. Thoroughly knead, integrating all ingredients with your hands. Makes about 3 cups.

Dehydrated Foods

Dehydrated foods make great snacks for work, travel, and kids' lunches. They help you lose weight much more easily because they offer taste satisfaction without a lot of calories. For example, Spicy Kale Chips (this page) are very low in calories and exceptionally high in nutrients such as calcium, magnesium, and vitamin K. Flax Crackers (page 205) and Awesome Corn Crackers (page 207) make wonderful snacks or accompaniment to meals and offer bursts of flavor along with fiber, enzymes, and an abundance of nutrients. It doesn't take much time to prepare them, and the rewards are great.

You'll notice that the dehydration temperature is 105 degrees for almost all dehydrated foods, which preserves nutrients, vitamins, and enzymes. There are a number of schools of thought as to what is the best temperature (between 105 and 118 degrees) to preserve the most enzymes and vitamins. When in doubt, choose the lower temperature setting on your dehydrator. (If you need a dehydrator, see Appendix A.)

Spicy Kale Chips

Kale is rich in lutein and zeaxanthin—two carotenoids that protect the cells from the damaging effects of free radicals and the eyes from developing age-related macular degeneration and cataracts.

> 1 bunch curly kale
> ¼ cup apple cider or coconut vinegar
> ¼ cup fresh lemon juice
> ¼ cup extra-virgin olive oil
> Pinch of cayenne pepper or red pepper flakes
> 2 tsp. garlic, minced or pressed
> ½ tsp. Celtic sea salt

Wash the kale and then cut it into 3-inch-long strips and set aside to dry.

Add vinegar, lemon juice, olive oil, and cayenne pepper or red pepper flakes to a blender and process on high speed until well combined. Pour the marinade into a bowl. Then dip the kale leaves in the marinade one at a time and massage the marinade into the leaf. Shake off excess marinade and place kale pieces on dehydrator P-Flexx sheets. Sprinkle with garlic and sea salt, and dehydrate for 4 to 8 hours at 105 degrees or until crisp. (Chips will get smaller as they dry.)

These chips are so delicious I'll bet you won't have many left to store. Makes about 4 trays of chips.

Broccoli-Carrot Crackers

Broccoli is rich in vitamin C as well as dietary fiber; it also contains many nutrients with potent anticancer properties, such as diindolylmethane and small amounts of selenium. And it contains the compound glucoraphanin, which is converted into the anticancer phytonutrient sulforaphane.

1½ pounds of broccoli (you can use the stems)
1 cup carrot pulp
1 medium sweet onion, cut into chunks
1 cup raw tahini
1 tsp. Celtic sea salt
2–3 pitted dates

Place broccoli in the food processor and process until shredded. Scoop this mixture into a bowl. Add the chunks of onion to the food processor and process until in small pieces; add to the bowl, along with the carrot pulp. Blend together the tahini, salt, and dates. Add this mixture to the vegetables in the bowl and mix well with your hands. Form into patties about 3 inches in diameter on dehydrator P-Flexx sheets. Dehydrate 8–10 hours and then turn them over carefully; dehydrate another 8–10 hours or until completely dry. Makes about 27 crackers.

Flax Crackers

Flaxseeds are rich in alpha-linolenic acid (ALA)—a type of plant-derived omega-3 fatty acid, similar to those found in fish such as salmon. Benefits of flaxseed as shown in many studies include lowering LDL cholesterol. Other benefits show that flaxseeds may help lower blood triglycerides and blood pressure. It may also keep platelets from becoming sticky, therefore reducing the risk of a heart attack.

2 cups flaxseeds
1 red bell pepper
1 carrot
½ cup sun-dried tomatoes
2 cups fresh tomatoes
Juice of 1 lemon
1 clove of fresh garlic
1 Tbsp. shoyu, tamari, or Braggs liquid aminos or 1–2 tsp. Celtic sea salt

Blend all ingredients together in a food processor. Add water if the batter is too dry. Press mixture flat onto a P-Flexx sheet into a large square that covers the sheet. Make sure that the mixture stands only about ⅛-inch high. The thicker the cracker, the chewier it is and the longer it takes to dry. With a knife or spatula, score the batch to the size you'd like before dehydrating. (A typical square is 3x3.) Dehydrate around 105 degrees overnight; flip over once one side is dry. Dehydrate until completely dry. Store in an airtight container. Makes about 27 crackers.

Nan's Carrot Curry Flax Krax

½–1 cup ground golden flaxseeds
1 cup warm water
1½ cup carrot juice
½-inch-chunk ginger root
1–2 tsp. orange zest
1 garlic clove
½ tsp. Celtic sea salt
1 Tbsp. onion, chopped
1 tsp. dried cilantro

Soak flaxseed for 2 or more hours. While seeds are soaking, juice carrots to get 1½ cups juice. Pour juice in a blender or food processor. Add all the other ingredients and blend until well combined. Batter should be the consistency of pancake batter. Add water as needed if it is too dry. Pour onto a P-Flexx tray. Score into desired cracker size. Dry at 105 degrees until crisp and breaks easily into pieces. Makes approximately 12 crackers.

Nan's Zesty Green Berry Krax

1 cup green grapes
1 cup blackberries
1 cup raspberries or strawberries
¼-inch-round-slice of organic lemon with skin
½-inch-chunk of ginger
1 large Granny Smith apple, chopped
2–3 Tbsp. barley green powder (your choice of brands)

Blend grapes in blender or food processor. Add the remaining ingredients and process until well combined. Dry soft and pliable for fruit roll-up options. Makes about 12 crackers.

Option: For super zesty, open up and sprinkle 3 teabags of Celestial Seasons Red Zinger or Berry Zinger herbal tea into the mixture.

Veggie Nut Crackers

1½ cups almonds, soaked overnight
1½ cups sunflower seeds, soaked 1–2 hours
1 cup pumpkin seeds, soaked 1–2 hours
7–8 cups veggie pulp (2 zucchini, 4 grated carrots or pulp
    leftover from juicing 4 carrots, 2 stalks celery, 2 red bell
    peppers, 1 small red onion chopped)
2 small Roma tomatoes, chopped
½ cup chopped fresh basil
½ cup chopped cilantro
Juice of ½ lemon
3 tsp. veggie seasoning
½ tsp. cayenne pepper
2–3 tsp. Celtic sea salt
2 tsp. dried dill

Drain water from nuts and seeds. Place almonds in a food processor, and add sunflower and pumpkin seeds; use the S blade and process until smooth in consistency. Set aside in a bowl.

Put all the chopped or grated veggies in the food processor; add the Roma tomatoes, basil, cilantro, and lemon juice.

Put the veggie mixture in with the nuts and seed mixture and combine well. Add spices and mix well.

Spread over P-Flexx sheets ⅓-inch thick, and score before dehydrating. Dehydrate for 16–20 hours at 105 degrees. Time will vary. Makes about 36 crackers.

Awesome Corn Crackers

½ cup golden flaxseeds, soaked 4–8 hours in 2 cups purified water
½ cup raw almonds, soaked, covered, 8 hours in purified water
2 cups fresh corn cut off the cob (about 6 ears of corn)
2 Tbsp. ground cumin
2 Tbsp. chopped sweet onion
1–2 tsp. Celtic sea salt

Blend flaxseeds and almonds in a food processor; add the other ingredients and process until mixture reaches consistency of pancake batter. Spoon about 1 tablespoon of batter onto the P-Flexx sheets and swirl with a spoon until it's a thin round layer, or cover about four P-Flexx sheets with batter spread very thin. Dehydrate 10–20 hours, depending on desired crispness. If you have covered the P-Flexx sheets, you can cut crackers to the shape desired when dry. You can also cut into strips for salads. Makes about 36 crackers.

Tomato Flat Bread

Whole-oat groats are a bigger grain than whole-wheat kernels. They contain vitamin E, several B vitamins, calcium, magnesium, and potassium. Oats also have some of the trace minerals selenium, copper, zinc, iron, and manganese.

1 cup almonds, soaked overnight
2 cups wheat berries or oat groats, soaked overnight
1 clove garlic
1 cup ground flaxseeds
1 cup tomato puree (made from fresh tomatoes)
1 cup water

The night before, soak almonds and grain (separately). When you are ready to make the bread, drain each. In food processor, mix the garlic and almonds until well ground. Place in large bowl. Put wheat or oat groats in processor and mix until a mash is created. Do not over-process once you reach that stage. Put in the bowl with the almonds and garlic. Add flaxseeds and stir until well combined. Add tomato puree and water; mix well. Spread on over two P-Flexx sheets about ¼-inch thick. Score to desired size. Dehydrate for 1 hour at 140 degrees. Reduce heat to 105 degrees and continue to dry for 8 more hours or until it reaches the desired dryness. Makes about 18 crackers.

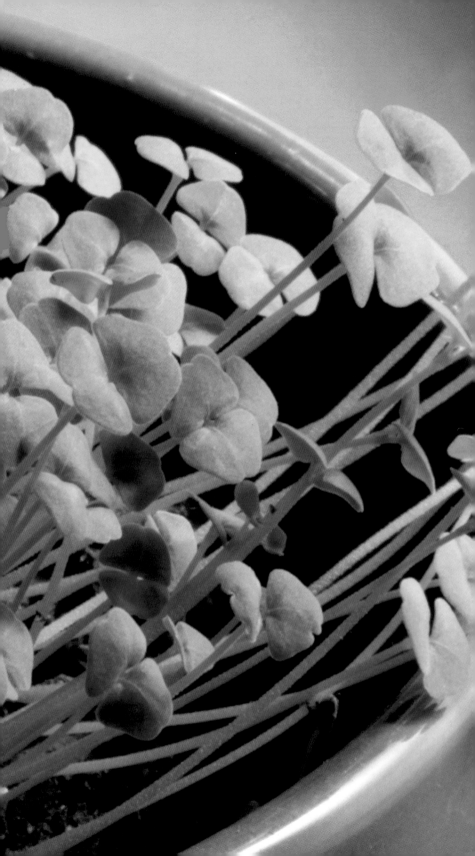

Main Courses

Cherie's Nut Burgers

Eating about a handful of pecans each day may play a role in protecting the nervous system, according to an animal study published in *Current Topics in Nutraceutical Research*.[8] Organic pecans are a good buy because pecan trees tend to be sprayed frequently with herbicides and miticides (pesticides that kills mites).

½ cup pecans or walnuts
¼ cup sunflower seeds
¼ cup hemp seeds
½ cup chia or flaxseeds (grind well)
½ cup sun-dried tomatoes, soaked 1 hour, drained and sliced
1 Tbsp. ginger, peeled and minced
2-3 cloves fresh garlic, pressed or minced
1 tsp. Celtic sea salt
2 carrots, chopped
1 stalk celery, chopped
½ cup red or yellow pepper, stemmed, seeded, chopped
½ cup zucchini, chopped
¼–½ cup dates, pitted and chopped
¼ sweet onion, chopped
¼ cup chopped parsley
1 Tbsp. fresh lemon juice
1 Tbsp. fresh oregano or 1 tsp. dried
1 Tbsp. water

Process the nuts and sunflower seeds in a food processor until ground fine. Add the hemp seeds and grind thoroughly. Set aside in a large bowl. Add the chia or flaxseeds to the ground nut and seed mixture; stir to mix.

Process the sun-dried tomatoes, ginger, garlic, and salt in the food processor. Add the carrots, celery, bell pepper, zucchini, dates, onion, parsley, lemon juice, oregano, and water. Process until well combined, but not mushy. Transfer the vegetable mixture to the ground nut and seed mixture.

Place half the mixture back in the food processor and pulse several times to mix well. Transfer to a new bowl. Repeat with remaining mixture.

Form patties. Dehydrate patties for 1 hour at 140 degrees. Reduce the temperature to 105 degrees and dehydrate for 4 hours or until top is dry. Flip the burgers and dehydrate another 4 hours or until as dry as desired. Serve with Healthy Raw Ketchup (page 200) and a slice of Tomato Flat Bread (page 207), as desired. Makes about 36 burgers.

Sunny Delight Enchiladas With Corn Tortillas

5 ears of corn with kernels cut off the cob
2 Tbsp. psyllium husk (not seed)
Purified water as needed
Nan's Sunflower Pate (page 213)
Nutty Cheese Sauce (page 202)

Place the corn and psyllim husk in a food processor and blend until smooth; add water as needed. Batter should be about the consistency of pancake batter. Place large spoonfuls of batter on dehydrator P-Flexx sheets. Using a spoon, swirl batter in a circular motion to shape into rounds to your desired tortilla size. Dehydrate about 4 hours at 105 degrees. Flip tortillas and dehydrate another 2 hours or until no longer wet yet soft and easy to roll. Don't leave in the dehydrator too long, or the tortillas will get hard. If that happens, you can make tostadas. Makes 16–20 tortillas.

To assemble tortillas:

Arrange tortillas on counter or breadboard. Top each tortilla with about 1 tablespoon of Nan's Sunflower Pate. Place a tablespoon of Nutty Cheese Sauce or guacamole on top of the filling; roll each tortilla into an enchilada style roll. It can be served with salsa or guacamole, as desired.

Chef Avi Dalene's Green Tortillas

It's nice to have some tortilla shells on hand for a variety of uses. This recipe can be used for chips, wraps, taquitos, burritos, and quesadillas. (See Appendix A for Chef Avi's *Raw Foods Recipe* DVD for these variations.) This recipe can be made in advance; the tortillas will keep in a sealed container in the refrigerator for several weeks.

> 1 cup chia seeds, unsoaked
> 4 cups zucchini (either with skins or peeled)
> 1 yellow or red bell pepper (red bell pepper will produce
>   darker tortilla color)
> 1 tsp. coriander
> 1 tsp. cumin
> 1 tsp. quality mineralized salt (Celtic sea or Himalayan salt)
> Jalapeño pepper to taste (green jalapeño peppers are unripe)
>   or a pinch of dried red pepper flakes
> ¼ cup young Thai coconut water (optional)
> 2 Tbsp. fresh lime juice (optional)
> 2 tsp. ultimate clear agave nectar (optional)

Using a high-speed blender, grind chia seeds into fine powder and set aside.

Place the zucchini, bell pepper, coriander, cumin, salt, jalapeño, and pepper into a high-speed blender and process until smooth. Add ground chia powder to mixture in high-speed blender and mix gently to dough/paste consistency.

If using, add young Thai coconut water, lime juice, and ultimate clear agave nectar (may need more or less) and mix until well combined.

Divide into 10 equal portions if making large tortillas, or 40 equal portions if making taquitos. Spread onto P-Flexx dehydrator sheets. Starting at one corner, add the mixture to the appropriate thickness and shape into tortillas. Make them about ¼-inch thick. Continue over the entire P-Flexx sheets until all the batter is used.

Dehydrate at 115 degrees for about 5 hours, or until desired dryness is reached. (They should be dry but flexible and soft. Do not over-dehydrate, or they will be hard.) Let set for several hours until you are ready to use them.

When dehydrating, if the tortillas get too crisp, dampen them slightly by spritzing them with a bit of good quality water. Also, the tortillas can be placed in the dehydrator to crisp up if they become moist while in storage.

Yields about 2½ dehydrator trays and makes 10 large tortillas, 40 taquito wraps, or some combination of the two.

Gourmet Pesto Pizza With Raw Buckwheat Groat Pizza Dough

This recipe for pizza dough also makes a delicious Italian Buckwheat cracker.

    2 cups sprouted buckwheat groats
    1-2 garlic cloves, chopped
    ¾ cup finely grated carrots (or use carrot pulp)
    ¾ cup soaked flaxseeds (soak overnight; they'll expand to
        about 1½ cups) or use ground flaxseeds and extra water
    ½ cup extra-virgin olive oil
    1 Tbsp. Italian seasonings (or fresh herbs to taste)
    1-2 tsp. Celtic sea salt
    Water as needed (usually ½-1 cup)
    1-1½ cups Raw Pesto Sauce (page 202)

Mix all ingredients together in a food processor. Start with buckwheat groats and garlic, followed by the rest of the ingredients. Coat a dehydrator sheet with a small amount of olive oil and scoop batches of dough (about a heaping tablespoon each) onto dehydrator sheets, swirling each scoop with a spoon to make rounds. You can make large pizza rounds (about 6 inches in diameter)—or you can make smaller individual rounds (about 3 inches in diameter). The smaller rounds are easier to serve and eat. Press out the dough evenly to about ⅛- to ¼-inch thick by patting the top with your fingertips or swirling with a spoon. If it gets too sticky, dip your fingers into some water to which you add a little olive oil. Once dough is pressed out evenly, dehydrate at 105-115 degrees for about 7 hours. Flip the crackers and dry another 7-10 hours or until crust is completely dry and crisp. (It should be crunchy for the best-tasting cracker.) To speed the drying process, transfer to the mesh rack. Use a spatula when lifting dough, and be careful when transferring it not to break the crackers. Makes 36 crackers.

Top with Raw Pesto Sauce. You can also top with Nutty Cheese Sauce (page 202) or Marinara Sauce (page 202).

NOTE: To sprout buckwheat, soak 1 cup raw buckwheat groats for about 2 hours; it will expand to about 2 cups. Drain and rinse well. Place on counter in a colander covered with a lightweight dishtowel or in a sprouter for one day. Rinse several times while sprouting. (If you don't have time to sprout, you can use buckwheat that has been soaked for 2 hours.)

NOTE: If crust is very dry and stored in a cool dry, airtight container, it can be kept fresh for several months.

Raw Zucchini Noodles With Marinara Sauce

    6 to 8 firm zucchini and/or yellow crookneck squash
    1 cup Marinara Sauce (page 202)
    Fresh basil, chopped, to taste (optional)
    Avocado slices (optional)

Use a vegetable spiral slicer or spirooli to make thin, long noodles out of zucchini. If possible, make zucchini noodles about six hours before serving, and let noodles sit in a bowl, uncovered, at room temperature, which can improve their texture.

Pour Marinara Sauce over the noodles, give the noodles and sauce a good toss, and serve. Top with chopped fresh basil and/or slices of avocado. Serves 3 to 4.

You can also use Raw Pesto Sauce (page 202). Or you can make my favorite—a simple pasta dish of zucchini noodles tossed with several tablespoons of extra-virgin olive oil, 2-3 cloves of pressed garlic, ¼ cup halved sun-dried olives, and ¼ cup chopped fresh basil. Sprinkle with salt, to taste, and serve.

Nan's Sunflower Pate

Sunflower seeds are an excellent source of vitamin E, the body's primary fat-soluble antioxidant. Vitamin E has significant anti-inflammatory effects that result in the reduction of symptoms in asthma, osteoarthritis, and rheumatoid arthritis, conditions where free radicals and inflammation play a big role.

3 cups sunflower seeds, soaked 8 to 12 hours; rinse and sprout about 4 hours
1 cup fresh lemon juice
½ cup scallions, chopped
¼-½ cup raw tahini
¼ cup liquid aminos or shoyu
2-4 slices red onion, cut into chunks
4-6 Tbsp. parsley, chopped
2-3 medium cloves garlic
½ tsp. cayenne pepper
1-2 Tbsp. ginger, chopped
1 tsp. ground cumin

Blend all ingredients in food processor until all the ingredients are smooth and creamy. This mixture should be on the thick side rather than thin. Add a bit of water as needed. Makes 7-8 cups.

Mock "Salmon" Pate

2 cups walnuts
2 carrots, grated, or use carrot pulp
2 ribs celery
1 large red bell pepper
2 green onions
1 large handful fresh parsley
½-1 tsp. Celtic sea salt
Raw Almond Mayo (page 203)
Almond slivers or slices (optional)

In a food processor, mix all ingredients together until smooth. Serve on a bed of lettuce with a dollop of Raw Almond Mayo or use as filling for stuffed tomatoes or stuffed avocados. Top with almond slivers or slices. Serves 6-8.

Marinated Collard Greens

Collard leaves are an excellent source of calcium and a fairly good source of magnesium and vitamin K, making this dish outstanding for healthy bones.

    4 Tbsp. extra-virgin olive oil
    Juice of 1 to 2 lemons
    1-2 cloves garlic, finely minced
    1 bunch fresh collard greens, washed; remove tough stems
        and trim out center vein

Place extra-virgin olive oil, lemon juice, and garlic in a small bowl and whisk together. Set aside.

Place collard leaves in large rectangular dish, alternating the direction of the leaves as you overlap and stack them. Pour in olive oil mixture, coating all leaves. Set aside for 3 hours before serving. Serves 10-12.

Almond Roulade

    Marinated Collard Greens (this page)
    Almond Filling (page 203)

Take collard greens and spread 2-3 tablespoons Almond Filling on one side of each leaf. Roll each collard leaf, forming roulade. Repeat this process, using up all Almond Filling and collard greens. Cut each roulade in half or thirds and serve one or two per person. Serves 10-12.

Almond Falafel

    3 cups almonds, soaked
    1½ cups sunflower seeds, soaked
    Juice of 2 lemons
    4 cloves garlic, finely chopped
    ½ cup raw tahini
    1½ Tbsp. curry
    3 cups of greens such as parsley, cilantro, or kale, finely
        chopped (use food processor or finely mince)

Soak nuts and seeds for several hours. Put drained, soaked almonds in food processor and chop fine. Set aside in a medium bowl. Process the soaked sunflower seeds and put in the bowl, adding lemon juice. Add garlic, tahini, curry, and greens. Mix everything together and massage with hands. Shape into small patties and serve fresh, or dehydrate at 105 degrees for 4-5 hours. Serve with the Sunflower Dill Sauce (page 198). Makes 6 servings.

Dolmas

20-24 collard leaves or grape leaves in season
1 cup apple-cider vinegar
2 Tbsp. extra-virgin olive oil
2 Tbsp. Celtic sea salt

Marinate leaves 3-6 hours in vinegar, olive oil, and salt. Make a V-cut at the end of each leaf, roll 2 cut ends up, place Zucchini Hummus (this page) inside, then tuck sides and roll up. Makes 20-24.

Zucchini Hummus

2 medium zucchini
2 tsp. olive oil
4 garlic cloves, 1 tsp. Celtic sea salt, or 1 tsp. dulse flakes
½ cup lemon or lime juice
½ cup sesame seeds
½ cup tahini
⅛ tsp. cayenne
1 tsp. paprika
1 tsp. cumin

Blend zucchini, oil, and garlic in food processor. Add remaining ingredients and blend. Serves 10-12.

Mango Salsa

3 cups tomatoes, diced
3 cups fresh mango, diced
½ cup onion, minced
½ cup cilantro, chopped
2 limes, juiced
1 garlic clove, minced
1 tsp. jalapeño, minced
½ tsp. Celtic sea salt

Mix all ingredients in a bowl and let the flavors mingle for at least 1 hour before serving. Serves 10.

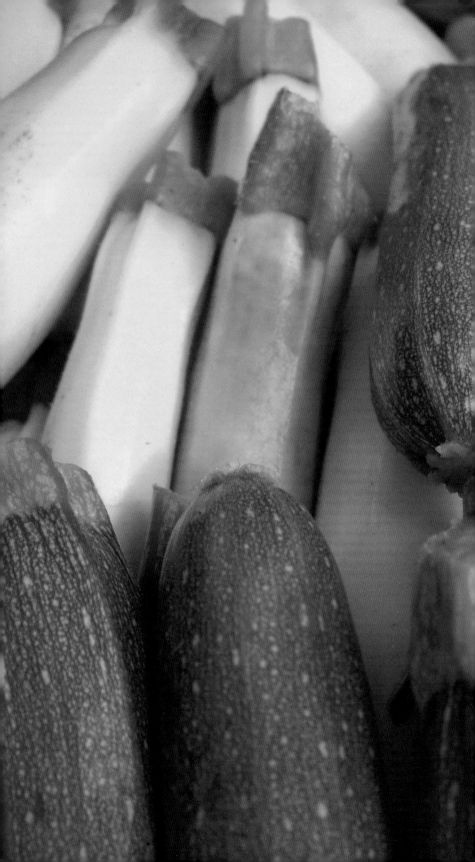

Cooked Food Recipes With Raw Foods

I've included some of my favorite cooked food recipes to give you an idea of how to include raw foods with cooked foods and increase your living foods intake.

Squash and Arugula Enchiladas

Delicata squash is my favorite in this recipe. It features yellow skin with green stripes on an oblong shape. A ¾-cup portion contains just 30 calories, so it's a great choice if you want to lose weight. It's also a good source of vitamin C and carotenes. Adding arugula or watercress gives you an example of combining cooked and living food.

2 delicata squash, 1 acorn squash, or ¼ butternut squash (other winter squash, sweet potatoes, or yams can be substituted)
1 cup brown rice, cooked
1 Tbsp. virgin coconut oil
4–6 tortillas (sprouted whole grain, spelt, or gluten free)
½–1 cup arugula, chopped
Salt and pepper to taste

Bake the delicata squash in a preheated oven set at 400 degrees for 30 minutes or until tender but not soft. Add water about an inch deep to the baking pan, and the squash cooks faster. While the squash is baking, cook the rice. (If you want meat in this dish, you can reduce the rice to ½ cup and add ½ pound of cooked ground meat.) When the squash is tender, remove from the oven and cut in half. If you are not using delicata squash, scoop out the seeds and peel; however, if you are using delicata and the skin is tender, you don't need to peel. Cut the squash in chunks and mix with rice; add seasoning to taste and set aside; keep warm.

In a large skillet, heat the oil. Heat the tortillas one at a time until warm and slightly browned, but be careful not to overcook or they will get crisp and won't roll into an enchilada. Spoon 2–3 tablespoons of the squash-rice mixture into the center of each tortilla and spread from one end to the other. Add arugula to the top of that mixture, adding salt and pepper to taste, and roll each side toward the center. Serve hot. Serves 4–6.

Carrot Sauce With Asparagus and Fresh Peas Over Rice

1 cup brown rice or quinoa
1½ cups carrot juice (about 8–11 carrots)
½ cup raw cashews
2 Tbsp. white or yellow miso
1 pound fresh asparagus
½ cup fresh or frozen peas
2 scallions, chopped
¼ cup marinated sun-dried tomato halves, thinly sliced
2 cloves garlic, pressed
3 Tbsp. fresh basil, finely chopped

Cook brown rice or quinoa according to directions.

While rice or quinoa is cooking, combine the carrot juice, cashews, and miso in a blender or food processor, blending on high until the cashews are no longer gritty and the mixture is smooth and creamy. Snap off the tops of the asparagus. Cut the tender upper portion into 1-inch pieces. In a medium-size skillet, combine the carrot juice mixture and asparagus. Bring to a boil and then reduce the heat to simmer, stirring occasionally for 2–3 minutes. Add the peas and simmer until the asparagus is just tender, about 2 minutes. Add the scallions, sun-dried tomatoes, and garlic, mixing well; simmer for 1–2 minutes. Remove the sauce from the heat.

Divide the rice or quinoa in 4 portions. Top each portion with about ¼ of the sauce and sprinkle chopped basil on top of each portion. Serves 4.

Nicole's Stuffed Acorn Squash

1 acorn squash
½ cup grass-fed ground turkey
¼ cup quinoa
1–2 garlic cloves, pressed
1 tsp. dried basil
½–1 tsp. Celtic sea salt
½ tsp. cumin
½ tsp. paprika
Broccoli-Cauliflower Slaw (page 197)
Red bell pepper strips

Bake the acorn squash at 400 degrees for 20 minutes. Remove from oven; cut squash in half and scoop out seeds. Return to oven and bake for 25 minutes, or until tender. Adding a little water to the baking pan will speed the baking process.

While the squash is baking, cook the ground turkey and quinoa in separate pans. When cooked, scoop the turkey and quinoa into a bowl and add the basil, salt, cumin, and paprika. Stir until well combined. Scoop half the mixture into each half of the acorn squash. Top each squash with a scoop of Broccoli-Cauliflower Slaw and several red bell pepper strips. Serves 2.

Nicole's Butternut Squash Soup

1 butternut squash, baked
1 cup coconut milk
¼ cup carrots, cooked
¼ cup celery, cooked
1 tsp. curry
1 tsp. cumin
½ tsp. cinnamon
Fresh basil, chopped, for garnish

Scoop the squash out of the skin. Add all the ingredients to the blender and puree. Pour into bowls and serve as soon as possible. Garnish with fresh chopped basil. Serves 3–4.

Lentil-Spinach Skillet Dinner

2 cups lentils
1 cup quinoa
2 Tbsp. virgin coconut oil
1 cup onion, chopped
2-3 carrots, chopped
2 cloves garlic, minced
2 Tbsp. ginger, chopped
2 lbs. fresh spinach, washed and dried
1-2 tsp. Celtic sea salt, to taste

Steam lentils according to instructions. Prepare quinoa according to instructions.

In a large skillet, melt coconut oil; add onions and carrots and sauté for about 5 minutes or until onion is translucent and carrots are tender. Turn to low heat. Add garlic and ginger; sauté for about 3 minutes. Place cooked lentils in skillet and mix well. Add spinach to the top and cover with a lid. Steam about 4 to 5 minutes, or until spinach is just slightly wilted. Serve over cooked quinoa, with salt to taste. Serves 3–4.

Cashew Mushroom Loaf

2 Tbsp. virgin coconut oil
1 small onion, chopped
2 garlic cloves, crushed
8 oz. cashews
4 oz. bread crumbs
3 medium parsnips, cooked and mashed
½ tsp. dried rosemary
½ tsp. thyme
1 tsp. Celtic sea salt
8 oz. fresh mushrooms, chopped
Hot water as needed

Preheat oven to 350 degrees. Heat 1 tablespoon oil and sauté onion and garlic until soft. Grind the cashews. In a medium to large bowl, mix ground cashews with breadcrumbs. Mix in the mashed parsnips and herbs. Add cooked onion mixture, making sure to scrape all juices into bowl. Add salt and mix. Add 1 tablespoon oil to pan and sauté mushrooms until soft. Grease a loaf pan. Press in half the cashew mixture. Add mushrooms and top with the remaining cashew mixture. Cover with foil and bake for 1 hour. Let stand for 10 minute before turning onto a plate and cutting into portions. Serves 4–6.

Healthy Desserts

Lemon Torte

1 cup cashews, soaked for 8 hours
2 lemons, zested
Juice of 2 lemons
2 Tbsp. pure maple syrup
1 orange, juiced
1 Tbsp. psyllium powder
Shortbread Crust (this page)

Blend all ingredients, except psyllium, in a blender until the mixture is the consistency of whipped cream. Fold in psyllium.

Pour into Shortbread Crust, cover with Saran Wrap, and freeze for at least 1 hour. Take out of freezer and refrigerate 30 minutes before serving. Serves 4.

Shortbread Crust

2½ cups shredded coconut
½ cup cashews, soaked 1 hour
2 Tbsp. honey

Put coconut in blender and start on low speed, then high. As well forms, slowly add cashews to crumbly stage. Then add honey. Use spatula if needed to blend. Blend until mixture heats a little bit.

Press crust in bottom and sides of 1 large or 4 small tart pans. Makes 4 small tarts or 1 large tart to use with your choice of fillings, such as Lemon Torte.

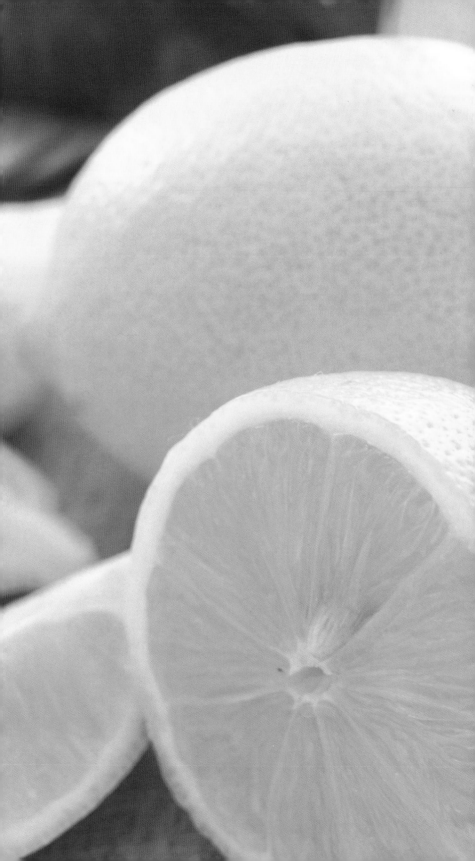

Summer Peach Parfait

- 7 peaches, peeled and thinly sliced
- 2 cups raw almonds, soaked in 3 cups purified water for 6–12 hours
- 4 Tbsp. raw almond butter
- ¼ cup honey or pure maple syrup
- ½ cup fresh orange juice
- 2 Tbsp. pure vanilla extract
- 2 tsp. cinnamon
- 4 tsp. nutmeg
- Pinch Celtic sea salt
- 2 pints blueberries (optional)

Blend 1 peeled peach and remaining ingredients, except blueberries. Add more orange juice as needed to aid in blending until a custard consistency is reached. In parfait glasses, layer peaches, custard, peaches, custard; top with blueberries (if using). Serves 8.

Appendix A

The Living Foods Resource Guide

Sign up for Cherie's free Juice Newsletter at www
.juiceladyinfo.com.

Cherie's websites

- www.juiceladyinfo.com—information on juicing and
  weight loss
- www.cheriecalbom.com—information about Cherie's
  websites
- www.sleepawaythepounds.com—information about the
  Sleep Away the Pounds program and products
- www.gococonuts.com—information about the Coconut
  Diet and coconut oil
- www.ultimatesmoothie.com—information about *The
  Ultimate Smoothie Book* and healthy smoothies

Other books by Cherie and John Calbom

These books can be ordered at any of the websites above or by calling
866.843.8935.

- Cherie Calbom, *The Juice Lady's Turbo Diet* (Siloam)
- Cherie Calbom, *The Juice Lady's Guide to Juicing for
  Health* (Penguin)
- Cherie Calbom with John Calbom, *Juicing, Fasting, and
  Detoxing for Life* (Grand Central Wellness)
- Cherie Calbom and John Calbom, *Sleep Away the
  Pounds* (Warner Wellness)
- Cherie Calbom, *The Wrinkle Cleanse* (Avery)
- Cherie Calbom and John Calbom, *The Coconut Diet*
  (Warner)
- Cherie Calbom, John Calbom, and Michael Mahaffey,
  The Complete Cancer Cleanse (Warner)
- Cherie Calbom, *The Ultimate Smoothie Book* (Warner)

Juicers

Find out the best juicers recommended by Cherie Calbom. Call 866-8GETWEL (866.843.8935) or visit www.juiceladyinfo.com.

Dehydrators

Find out the best dehydrators recommended by Cherie Calbom. Call 866-8GETWEL (866.843.8935) or visit www.juiceladyinfo.com.

Lymphasizer

To view the Swing Machine (lymphasizer), visit www.juiceladyinfo.com or call 866-8GETWEL (866.843.8935).

Veggie powders

To purchase or get information on Barley Max, Carrot Max, and Beet Max powders, call 866.843.8935. (These powders are ideal for when you travel or when you can't get juice.)

Virgin coconut oil

For more information on virgin coconut oil, go to www.gococonuts.com or call 866.843.8935. To save money, order larger sizes such as gallons or quarts, which you won't typically find in the stores.

Organic food delivered to you

Call Cherie at 866.843.8935 for more information about organic produce and grass-fed meat and dairy products that you can order delivered to your door.

Supplements

- Multivitamins and Citramins (multi-minerals) by Thorne Research: call 866.843.8935
- Digestive enzymes Ness Formula #4 and #16 are excellent to aid digestion. Taken between meals, they help clean up undigested proteins, fats, and carbs. With the addition of enzymes, you should notice that your hair and nails grow better. Call 866-8GETWEL (866.843.8935)
- Calcium Citrate or Calcium Citramate (contains both calcium citrate-malate and malic acid; offers good solubility and superb absorption when compared to other forms of calcium) by Thorne Research: call 866.843.8935

- Magnesium Citrate or Magnesium Citramate (as Magnesium Citrate-Malate and malic acid) by Thorne Research: call 866.843.8935
- Vitamin C with bioflavonoids or Buffered C Powder (contains ascorbic acid, calcium, magnesium, and potassium) by Thorne Research or Allergy Research: call 866.843.8935
- Vitamin D_3 (1,000 or 5,000 mg) by Thorne Research: call 866.843.8935

Colon cleanse products

Call 866.843.8935 for more information on Cherie's recommendations below.

- Medibulk by Thorne (psyllium powder, prune powder apple pectin)
- Blessed Herbs Colon Cleanse Kit: After years of eating standard food, it's quite common to build up a layer of mucoid plaque—hardened mucus-like material and food residue that can coat the gastrointestinal tract. Nutrients are absorbed through the intestinal wall. The plaque hinders our ability to absorb nutrients, which can lead to numerous health problems. This colon cleanse kit contains products that can pull the plaque from your intestinal wall and carry it out of your system—Digestive Stimulator, Toxin Absorber, glass shaker jar, and user guide and dosage calendar. Specify ginger or peppermint flavor. Cost: $89.50 less 5 percent discount, if you call and mention this book offer.

Internal Cleansing Kit

Blessed Herbs complete and comprehensive internal cleansing kit contains 18 items for a 21-day cleanse program with free colon cleanse kit. You get a free colon cleanse kit, along with Liver-Gallbladder Rejuvenator, Friendly Bacteria Replenisher, Parasite Cleanser, Lung Rejuvenator, Kidney and Bladder Rejuvenator, Blood and Skin Rejuvenator, and Lymph Rejuvenator, along with glass shaker jar and user guide and dosage calendar. Specify ginger or peppermint flavor. Cost $279, less 5 percent discount, if you call and mention this book offer.

If you want to read more about Blessed Herbs Cleansing Kits, go to my website www.juiceladyinfo.com. You will need to order via 866.843.8935 to get the discount, however.

Liver/gallbladder cleanse products

- S.A.T. by Thorne (milk thistle, artichoke, turmeric) along with Cysteplus (N-Acetyl-L-Cysteine) and Lipotropein (vitamins, minerals, L-Methionine, and herbs including dandelion, beet leaf, and black radish root)—call 866.843.8935
- Chinese herbal tinctures (4-part kit) to use with Cherie's Liver Detox Program—call 866.843.8935

Candida albicans cleanse products

- Friendly Bacteria Replenisher—visit www.juiceladyinfo .com
- Blessed Herbs Total Body Cleanse—visit www .juiceladyinfo.com or call 866.843.8935

Parasite cleanse products

- Large Para Cleanser 1 and 2 and Small Para Cleanser— visit www.juiceladyinfo.com
- Blessed Herbs Total Body Cleanse—visit www .juiceladyinfo.com or call 866.843.8935

Kidney cleanse herbs

- Blessed Herbs Kidney-Bladder Rejuvenator—call 866.843.8935

Heavy metal and toxic compounds cleanse products

For all these products, call 866.843.8935.

- Captomer by Thorne (Succinic acid from 100 mg DMSA)—chelates heavy metals
- Heavy Metal Support by Thorne—replaces important minerals and other nutrients lost during metal chelating
- Toxic Relief Booster by Thorne—nutrients designed to aid in metabolizing the increased amount of fat stored toxins released into the bloodstream during a cleanse
- Formaldehyde Relief by Thorne—provides nutrients necessary for detoxification of formaldehyde from new carpet and furniture outgassing, as well as compounds produced by Candida albicans or by alcohol metabolism

- Solvent Remover by Thorne—contains amino acids specific to solvent detoxification in the liver, as well as nutrients that help protect nerves from solvent damage
- Pesticide Protector by Thorne—aids in detoxification of chlorinated pesticides, organophosphates, carbamates, and pyrethrins

INFORMATION AND PRODUCTS FOR SPECIFIC DISORDERS

Sleep disorders and brain neurotransmitter and adrenal test kit

Testing neurotransmitters is the best way to determine if you have depletion in brain chemicals that could be causing sleep problems. Testing can be completed whether you are taking medications or not. You can determine if your neurotransmitters are out of balance by taking the Brain Wellness Program's Self Test. This is also the site for the Adrenal Test. Just go to www.Neurogistics.com and click "Get Started." Use the practitioner code SLEEP (all caps). You can order the program, which includes a urine in-home test that will yield a report on your neurotransmitter levels. And if you are fatigued and sense you may have low adrenal function, order the saliva test kit. You'll be given a customized protocol with guidelines for the right amino acids and supplements for you to take to help correct your imbalances. Or you can call 866.843.8935 for more information.

RECIPE PRODUCTS

The Smart Raw Food Method DVD with Chef Avi Dalene, MA

This DVD includes Chef Avi's Green Tortillas. Available at http://www .smartrawfood.com/eStore.html and Amazon.com.

NATUROPATHIC PHYSICIAN

Naturopathic physician Nina Walsh incorporates juicing, raw foods, and wild greens in her protocols. Below is her contact information.

Nina Walsh, ND
Flow Natural Medicine
PHONE: 206.384.2414
E-MAIL: ninawalshnd@yahoo.com
WEBSITE: www.flowmedicine.com

Health Centers Utilizing Juice and Raw Foods Cleanse Programs

T HE FOLLOWING CENTERS offer a raw foods and/or juice detoxification program. Most of them offer nutritional classes, and some offer other health classes that address the emotional, mental, and spiritual aspects of health and renewal. Most of the centers also offer massage and colonics. It is best to contact the various centers to find out which one best fits your needs.

HealthQuarters Ministries
David Frahm, ND, Director
3620 W. Colorado Ave.
Colorado Springs, CO 80904
Phone: 719.593.8694
Fax: 719.531.7884
E-mail: healthqu@healthquarters.org
Web site: www.healthquarters.org

Hippocrates Institute
Brian and Anna Maria Clement, Directors
1443 Palmdale Ct.
West Palm Beach, FL 33411
Phone: 800.842.2125
Fax: 561.471.9464
E-mail: hippocrates@worldnet.att.net
Web site: www.hippocratesinstitute.org

Optimum Health Institute of Austin
Route 1 Box 339 J
Cedar Creek, TX 78612
Phone: 512.303.4817
Fax: 512.303.1239
E-mail: austin@optimumhealth.org
Website: www.optimumhealth.org

Optimum Health Institute of San Diego
6970 Central Ave.
Lemon Grove, CA 91945-2198
Phone: 800.993.4325
Fax: 619.589.4098
E-mail: optimum@optimumhealth.org
Website: www.optimumhealth.org

Sanoviv Medical Institute
Dr. Myron Wentz, Director
Playa de Rosarito, Km 39
Baja, California, Mexico
Phone: 800.726.6848
Fax: 801.954.7477
Website: www.sanoviv.com

Thrive Wellness Center
Monika Kinsman, Director
31459 Barben Road
Sedro Woolley, WA 98284
Phone: 206.334.7111
Website: www.generationthrive.com/wellness-center

We Care
Susana and Susan Lombardi, Directors
18000 Long Canyon Rd.
Desert Hot Springs, CA 92241
Phone: 800.888.2523
Fax: 760.251.5399
E-mail: info@wecarespa.com
Web site: www.wecarespa.com

Notes

1—THE LIVING FOODS REVOLUTION

1. Mary Enig and Sally Fallon, "The Oiling of America," *Nexus Magazine*, December 1998/January 1999, as viewed at http://alpha-health-plus.com/ Oiling_of_America-_History_of_Fats_&_Oils_03.html (accessed March 8, 2011).

2. C. V. Felton, D. Crook, M. J. Davies, and M. F. Oliver, "Dietary Polyunsaturated Fatty Acids and Composition of Human Aortic Plaques," *Lancet* 344, no. 8931 (October 29, 1994): 1195–1196.

3. UT Health Science Center news release, "New Analysis Suggests 'Diet Soda Paradox'—Less Sugar, More Weight," June 14, 2005, http://www.uthscsa .edu/hscnews/singleformat2.asp?newID=1539 (accessed March 8, 2011).

4. Internet Movie Database, "Synopsis for *Super Size Me* (2004)," http://www .imdb.com/title/tt0390521/synopsis (accessed March 8, 2011).

5. McDonalds.com, "Chicken McNuggets: Nutrition," http://www.mcdonalds .com/us/en/food/full_menu/chicken/mcnuggets.html (accessed March 8, 2011).

6. Mercola.com, "The Chicken Which Should Be Banned: Dr. Mercola's Comments," November 8, 2010, http://articles.mercola.com/sites/articles/ archive/2010/11/08/do-you-have-any-idea-of-the-chemicals-used-in-fast -food-chicken.aspx (accessed March 8, 2011).

7. Sally Fallon Morell, "Dirty Secrets of the Food Processing Industry," presentation given at the annual conference of Consumer Health of Canada, March 2002, http://www.westonaprice.org/modern-foods/567- dirty-secrets -of-the-food-processing-industry.html (accessed March 8, 2011).

8. As referenced in Sally Fallon, "Puffed Grains and Breakfast Cereals: Should We Eat Them?" NourishedMagazine.com, December 2008, http://editor .nourishedmagazine.com.au/articles/puffed-grains-should-we-eat-them (accessed March 8, 2011).

9. "How to Be a Good Wife," in the 1950's American High School Home Economics Textbook, referenced in Roobix Coob, "A Woman's Role in the 1950s," http://www.colorado.edu/AmStudies/lewis/1025/women1950s.pdf (accessed March 8, 2011).

10. Mary Dixon Lebeau, "At 50, TV Dinner Is Still Cookin'," CSMonitor.com, November 10, 2004, http://www.csmonitor.com/2004/1110/p11s01-lifo.html (accessed March 8, 2011).

11. A. Blair, S. H. Zahm, N. E. Pearce, E. F. Heineman, and J. F. Fraumeni Jr., "Clues to Cancer Etiology From Studies of Farmers," *Scandinavian Journal of Work, Environment and Health* (Helsinki) 18, no. 4 (1992): 209–215.

12. Joseph Mercola, "McDonald's and Biophoton Deficiency," Mercola .com, August 21, 2002, http://articles.mercola.com/sites/articles/ archive/2002/08/21/biophoton.aspx (accessed March 8, 2011).

13. John Switzer, "Bio-Photon Nutrition and Wild Green Energy Cocktails for Optimal Health (English)," May 21, 2009, http://www.ein-langes-leben

.de/index.php?option=com_content&view=article&id=186:bio-photon
-nutrition-and-wild-energy-cocktails-for-optimal-health-english&catid=32:
english&Itemid=99 (accessed March 8, 2011).

14. Marco Bischof, "Humans Emit Biophotons—the Light of Our Cells,"
HeartSpring.net, January 30, 2011, http://heartspring.net/meditation_
biophoton.html (accessed March 8, 2011).

15. Arthur M. Baker, "Raw Fresh Produce vs. Cooked Food," RawFoodHowTo
.com, http://www.rawfoodhowto.com/raw-fresh-produce-vs-cooked.cfm
(accessed March 8, 2011).

16. Timothy J. A. Key, Margaret Thorogood, Paul N. Appleby, and Michael
L. Burr, "Dietary Habits and Mortality in 11,000 Vegetarians and Health
Conscious People: Results of a 17-Year Follow Up," *British Medical
Journal* 313, no. 7060 (September 28, 1996): 775, http://www.bmj.com/
content/313/7060/775.full (accessed March 8, 2011).

17. Secretariat.com, "Secretariat History," http://www.secretariat.com/
secretariat-history/ (accessed March 8, 2011); Secretariat.com, "Wood
Memorial," http://www.secretariat.com/past-performances/wood-memorial/
(accessed March 8, 2011).

18. Steven Cesari, *Clarity* (Charleston, SC: Advantage, 2010), 35.

2—Juicing for a Healthy Lifestyle

1. Jane E. Brody, "Even Benefits Don't Tempt Us to Vegetables," *New
York Times*, October 4, 2010, http://www.nytimes.com/2010/10/05/
health/05brody
.html?_r=1 (accessed January 30, 3011).

2. Joseph Mercola, "The Best and Worst Vegetables to Eat," Mercola
.com, November 29, 2010, http://articles.mercola.com/sites/articles/
archive/2010/11/29/recommended-vegetable-list.aspx (accessed December
30, 2010).

3. Ibid.

4. Francesca L. Crowe et al., "Fruit and Vegetable Intake and Mortality
From Ischaemic Heart Disease: Results From the European Prospective
Investigation Into Cancer and Nutrition (EPIC)–Heart Study," *European
Heart Journal*, January 18, 2011, http://eurheartj.oxfordjournals.org/content/
early/2011/01/17/eurheartj.ehq465.abstract (accessed February 28, 2011).

5. NHS.uk, "Five a Day 'Saves Lives,'" http://www.nhs.uk/
news/2010/12December/Pages/five-a-day-saves-lives.aspx (accessed
February 28, 2011).

6. Patrice Carter, Laura J. Gray, Jacqui Troughton, Kamlesh Khunti, and
Melanie J. Davies, "Fruit and Vegetable Intake and Incidence of Type 2
Diabetes Mellitus: Systematic Review and Meta-Analysis," *British Medical
Journal* 341 (August 2010): http://www.bmj.com/content/341/bmj.c4229.full
(accessed March 8, 2011).

7. Diane Feskanich et al., "Vitamin K Intake and Hip Fractures in Women:
A Prospective Study," *American Journal of Clinical Nutrition* 69, no. 1
(January 1999): 74–79, http://www.ajcn.org/content/69/1/74.full (accessed
February 22, 2011).

8. Susanna C. Larsson, Leif Bergkvist, Ingmar Näslund, Jörgen Rutegård
and Alicja Wolk, "Vitamin A, Retinol, and Carotenoids and the Risk

of Gastric Cancer: A Prospective Cohort Study," *American Journal of Clinical Nutrition* 85, no. 2 (February 2007): 497–503, http://www.ajcn.org/content/85/2/497.full (accessed February 28, 2011).

9. Whfoods.com, "Garlic," http://www.whfoods.com/genpage.php?tname=foodspice&dbid=60 (accessed January 30, 2011).

10. Jeannelle Boyer and Rui Hai Liu, "Apple Phytochemicals and Their Health Benefits," *Nutrition Journal* 3, no. 5 (May 2004), http://www.nutritionj.com/content/3/1/5 (accessed March 9, 2011).

11. A. S. Kutama, I. Yusuf, and M. Hayatu, "Detection of Heat-Resistant Molds in Some Canned Fruit Juices Sold in Kano, Nigeria," *Bioscience Research Communications* 22, no. 4 (2010).

12. Morell, "Dirty Secrets of the Food Processing Industry."

13. Penny Fannin, "Mad Cow Disease Theory Challenged by Mark Purdey," *The Age* (Australia), April 24, 2001, http://www.mindfully.org/Farm/Mad-Cow-Mark-Purdey.htm (accessed March 9, 2011).

14. Fran Lowery, "Repeated Exposure to Pesticides Increases Alzheimer's Disease Risk," *Medscape Medical News*, May 19, 2010, http://www.medscape.com/viewarticle/722040 (accessed March 9, 2011).

15. PRNewswire.com, "How Much Do Fruits and Vegetables Really Cost?", February 3, 2011, http://www.prnewswire.com/news-releases/how-much-do-fruits-and-vegetables-really-cost-115223374.html (accessed March 9, 2011).

16. Alan Greene, "Five Easy Ways to Go Organic," *Eartheasy* (blog), *Organic Prescription*, January 28, 2009, http://eartheasy.com/blog/2009/01/five-easy-ways-to-go-organic/ (accessed March 9, 2011).

17. G. Carrera, J. Alary, M. J. Melgar, Y. Lamboeuf, and B. Pipy, "Metabolism and Cytotoxicity of Chlorpropham (CIPC) and Its Essential Metabolites in Isolated Rat Hepatocytes During a Partial Inhibition of Sulphation and Glucuronidation Reactions: A Comparative Study," *Archives of Environmental Contamination and Toxicology* 35, no. 1 (July 1998): 89–96.

18. Greene, "Five Easy Ways to Go Organic."

19. Environmental Working Group, "The Full List: 49 Fruits and Veggies," Shopper's Guide to Pesticides, http://www.foodnews.org/fulllist.php (accessed January 28, 2011).

20. Ibid.

21. Dan Shapley, "The New Dirty Dozen: 12 Foods to Eat Organic and Avoid Pesticide Residue," *The Daily Green News* (blog), Yahoo! Green, April 28, 2010, http://green.yahoo.com/blog/daily_green_news/332/the-new-dirty-dozen-12-foods-to-eat-organic-and-avoid-pesticide-residue.html (accessed March 9, 2011).

22. Environmental Working Group, "The Full List: 49 Fruits and Veggies."

23. As referenced in GoodFood World Staff, "Organics From Mexico—Are They Safe?", February 2, 2011, http://www.goodfoodworld.com/2011/02/organics-from-mexico-are-they-safe/ (accessed March 9, 2011).

3—Weight Loss on a Mission

1. As referenced in Antoaneta Sawyer, "Role of Probiotics and Prebiotics in the Modern Diet," Examiner.com, June 12, 2010, http://www.examiner.com/diets-in-milwaukee/role-of-probiotics-and-prebiotics-the-modern-diet (accessed March 9, 2011).

2. Lenka J. Zajic, "Raw Food Diet Study," *Iowa Source*, August 6, http://www .iowasource.com/food/lenkastudy_0806.html (accessed December 16, 2010).

3. National Weight Control Registry, "NWCR Facts," http://www.nwcr.ws/ Research/default.htm (accessed March 9, 2011).

4. "Dr. Oz's Top 5 Mistakes Dieters Make," posted by Norine Dworkin-McDaniel, ThatsFit.com, December 26, 2010, http://www.thatsfit .com/2010/12/26/dr-ozs-top-5-mistakes-dieters-make/ (accessed March 9, 2011).

5. Mark A. Pereira, Janis Swain, Allison B. Goldfine, Nader Rifai, and David S. Ludwig, "Effects of a Low-Glycemic Load Diet on Resting Energy Expenditure and Heart Disease Risk Factors During Weight Loss," *Journal of the American Medical Association* 292, no. 20 (November 24, 2004): 2482–2490.

6. *First for Women*, "Dr. Oz's #1 Fat Cure," January 10, 2011, 32–35.

7. Adein Cassidy et al., "Plasma Adiponectin Concentrations Are Associated With Body Composition and Plant-Based Dietary Factors in Female Twins," *Journal of Nutrition* 139, no. 2 (February 2009): 353–358.

8. University of Nottingham, "Looking Good on Greens," press release, January 11, 2011, http://www.nottingham.ac.uk/news/pressreleases/2011/ january/lookinggoodongreens.aspx (accessed March 6, 2011).

9. ScienceDaily.com, "Brain Chemical Boosts Body Heat, Aids in Calorie Burn, UT Southwestern Research Suggests," July 7, 2010, http://www. sciencedaily .com/releases/2010/07/100706123015.htm (accessed March 6, 2011).

10. ScienceDaily.com, "Peppers May Increase Energy Expenditure in People Trying to Lose Weight," April 28, 2010, http://www.sciencedaily.com/ releases/2010/04/100427190934.htm (accessed December 28, 2010).

11. Judy Siegel, "Garlic Prevents Obesity," *Jerusalem Post*, October 30, 2001, 5.

12. Niki Fears, "Cranberries and Weight Loss," eHow.com, http://www.ehow .com/about_5417851_cranberries-weight-loss.html (accessed December 28, 2010).

13. *Woman's World*, "Slimming New Juice Cure," December 27, 2010, 18–19.

14. ScienceDaily.com, "Blueberries May Help Reduce Belly Fat, Diabetes Risk," April 20, 2009, http://www.sciencedaily.com/releases/2009/04/090419170112 .htm (accessed March 9, 2011).

15. *First for Women*, "Break the Yeast–Belly Fat Cycle," September 6, 2010, 30–31.

16. Ibid., 33.

17. Ulrich Harttig and George S. Bailey, "Chemoprotection by Natural Chlorophylls *in vivo*: Inhibition of Dibenzo[*a,l*]pyrene–DNA Adducts in Rainbow Trout Liver," *Carcinogenesis* 19, no. 7 (1998): 1323–1326.

18. Mercola.com, "The Truth About Candida Overgrowth," December 4, 2009, http://www.drmercola.info/2009/12/the-truth-about-candida-overgrowth/ (accessed March 9, 2011).

19. Anne M. Stark, "Eating Greens Every Day Keeps the Toxins Away," LLNL Community News, January 22, 2010, https://newsline.llnl.gov/_rev02/ articles/2010/jan/01.22.10-toxin.php (accessed March 6, 2011).

20. R. E. Ley, P. J. Turnbaugh, S. Klein, and J. I. Gordon, "Microbial Ecology: Human Gut Microbes Associated With Obesity," *Nature* 444, no. 7122 (December 21, 2006): 1022–1023.

21. Y. Kadooka et al., "Regulation of Abdominal Adiposity by Probiotics (Lactobacillus gasseri SBT2055) in Adults With Obese Tendencies in a Randomized Controlled Trial," *European Journal of Clinical Nutrition* 64, no. 6 (June 2010): 636–643.

22. Katherine Zeratsky, "Probiotics: Important for a Healthy Diet?", MayoClinic
.com, April 17, 2010, http://www.mayoclinic.com/health/probiotics/
AN00389 (accessed March 9, 2011).

23. D. O. Ogbolu, A. A. Oni, O. A. Daini, and A. P. Oloko, "*In Vitro* Antimicrobial Properties of Coconut Oil on Candida Species in Ibadan, Nigeria," *Journal of Medical Food* 10, no. 2 (June 2007): 384–387.

24. Joseph Mercola, "This Cooking Oil Is a Powerful Virus-Destroyer and Antibiotic…," Mercola.com, October 22, 2010, http://articles.mercola.com/
sites/articles/archive/2010/10/22/coconut-oil-and-saturated-fats-can-make
-you-healthy.aspx (accessed March 9, 2011).

25. Ibid.

26. Ibid.

27. *First for Women*, "Break the Yeast–Belly Fat Cycle," 31.

28. USAToday.com, "Study: 10 Minutes of Exercise Yields Hour-Long Effects," June 1, 2010, http://www.usatoday.com/news/health/weightloss/2010-06-01
-exercise-metabolism_N.htm (accessed March 9, 2011).

29. Ibid.

30. Cherie Calbom and John Calbom, *Sleep Away the Pounds* (New York: Warner Wellness, 2007).

31. Rob Stein, "Scientists Finding Out What Losing Sleep Does to a Body," *Washington Post*, October 9, 2005, http://www.washingtonpost.com/
wp-dyn/content/article/2005/10/08/AR2005100801405.html (accessed March 9, 2011).

32. Will Wilkoff, *Is My Child Overtired?* (New York: Fireside, 2000), 14.

33. Nanci Hellmich, "Sleep Loss (May) = Weight Gain: Healthy Weight Might Rest With Diet, Exercise and Sleep-Linked Hormones," *USA Today*, December 7, 2004, http://www.usatoday.com/educate/college/healthscience/
articles/20041212.htm (accessed March 10, 2011).

34. James E. Gangwisch, Dolores Malaspina, Bernadette Boden-Albala, and Steven B. Heymsfield, "Inadequate Sleep as a Risk Factor for Obesity: Analyses of the NHANES I," *Sleep* 28, no. 10 (2005): 1289–1296.

35. Colette Bouchez, "The Dream Diet: Losing Weight While You Sleep," WebMD.com, http://www.webmd.com/sleep-disorders/guide/lose-weight
-while-sleeping (accessed March 10, 2011).

36. John Easton, "Lack of Sleep Alters Hormones, Metabolism," *University of Chicago Chronicle*, December 2, 1999, http://chronicle.uchicago.edu/991202/
sleep.shtml (accessed March 10, 2011).

37. Bouchez, "The Dream Diet: Losing Weight While You Sleep."

38. Ibid.

39. Easton, "Lack of Sleep Alters Hormones, Metabolism."

40. Cherie Calbom and John Calbom, *Sleep Away the Pounds* (New York: Warner Wellness, 2007).

4—LIVING FOODS FOR THYROID AND ADRENAL HEALTH

1. Bodil-Cecilie Sondergaard, Svetlana Oestergaard, Claus Christiansen, Laszló B. Tankó, and Morten Asser Karsdal, "The Effect of Oral Calcitonin on Cartilage Turnover and Surface Erosion in an Ovariectomized Rat Model," *Arthritis and Rheumatism* 56, no. 8 (August 2007): 2647–2678.

2. Na Li, Donghong Wang, Yiqi Zhou, Mei Ma, Jian Li, and Zijian Wang, "Dibutyl Phthalate Contributes to Thyroid Receptor Antagonistic Activity in Drinking Water Processes," *Environmental Science and Technology* 44, no. 17 (September 1, 2010): 6863–6868.

3. Kellyn S. Betts, "Thyroid Insult: Flame Retardants Linked to Alterations in Pregnant Women's TSH Levels," *Environmental Health Perspectives* 118, no. 10 (October 2010): 445.

4. Rachel A. Heimeier, Biswajit Das, Daniel R. Buchholz, and Yun-Bo Shi, "The Xenoestrogen Bisphenol A Inhibits Postembryonic Vertebrate Development by Antagonizing Gene Regulation by Thyroid Hormone," *Endocrinology* 150, no. 6 (June 2009): 2964–2943.

5. Lyn Patrick, "Thyroid Disruption: Mechanisms and Clinical Implications in Human Health," *Alternative Medicine Review* 14, no. 4 (December 2009): 326–346.

6. *Environmental Health Perspectives*, "Stain Repellent Chemical Linked to Thyroid Disease in U.S. Adults," news release, January 21, 2010, http://ehp03.niehs.nih.gov/static/20100224c.action (accessed March 10, 2011).

7. Environmental Working Group, "44 Million Women at Risk of Thyroid Deficiency From Rocket Fuel Chemical," news release, October 4, 2006, http://www.ewg.org/release/44-million-women-risk-thyroid-deficiency -rocket-fuel-chemical (accessed March 10, 2011).

8. Craig Steinmaus, Mark D. Miller, and Robert Howd, "Impact of Smoking and Thiocyanate on Perchlorate and Thyroid Hormone Associations in the 2001–2002 National Health and Nutrition Examination Survey," *Environmental Health Perspectives* 115, no. 9 (September 2007): 1333–1338.

9. Ryan Robbins, "Are Nonstick Pans Linked to Thyroid Disease?", Bastyr University Health Tips, January 26, 2011, http://bastyr.edu/news/news .asp?NewsID=2272 (accessed March 10, 2011).

10. *Environmental Health Perspectives*, "Stain Repellent Chemical Linked to Thyroid Disease in U.S. Adults."

11. Robbins, "Are Nonstick Pans Linked to Thyroid Disease?"

12. R. L. Divi, H. C. Chang, and D. R. Doerge, "Anti-Thyroid Isoflavones From Soybean: Isolation, Characterization, and Mechanisms of Action," *Biochemical Pharmacology* 54, no. 10 (November 15, 1997): 1087–1096.

13. Mary Shomon, "Do Soy Products Negatively Affect Your Thyroid?", Thyroid -Info.com, http://www.thyroid-info.com/articles/soydangers.htm (accessed March 10, 2011).

14. P. Fort, N. Moses, M. Fasano, T. Goldberg, and F. Lifshitz, "Breast and Soy-Formula Feeding in Early Infancy and the Prevalence of Autoimmune Thyroid Disease in Children," *Journal of the American College of Nutrition* 9, no. 2 (April 1990): 164–167.

15. L. Kotze, R. Nisihara, S. Utiyama, G. Custodio Piovezan, and L. R. Kotze, "Thyroid Disorders in Brazilian Patients With Celiac Disease," *Journal of Clinical Gastroenterology* 40, no. 1 (January 2006): 33–36.

16. S. Pavelka, "Metabolism of Bromide and Its Interference With the Metabolism of Iodine," *Physiological Research* 53, Suppl. 1 (2004): S80–S90.

17. Ibid.

18. C. Pelletier, P. Imbeault, and A. Tremblay, "Energy Balance and Pollution by Organochlorines and Polychlorinated Biphenyls," *Obesity Reviews* 4, no. 1 (February 2003): 17–24.

19. TruthAboutSplenda.com, "Frequently Asked Questions," http://www.truthaboutsplenda.com/resources/faqs.html (accessed March 24, 2011).

20. Andrea McCreery, "How to Protect Yourself From Radiation Exposure," Life-Sources.com, March 17, 2011, http://www.life-sources.com/news/70/How-to-Protect-Yourself-from-Radiation-Exposure.html (accessed March 21, 2011).

21. Ahmet Koyua, Gokhan Cesura, Fehmi Ozgunera, Mehmet Akdoganb, Hakan Mollaoglua and Sukru Ozenc, "Effects of 900 MHz Electromagnetic Field on TSH and Thyroid Hormones in Rats," *Toxicology Letters* 157, nos. 3, 4 (July 2005): 257–262.

5—Living Foods for Detoxification

1. PollutionIssues.com, "Endocrine Disruption," http://www.pollutionissues.com/Ec-Fi/Endocrine-Disruption.html (accessed March 22, 2011).

2. Tracey J. Woodruff, Ami R. Zota, and Jackie M. Schwartz, "Environmental Chemicals in Pregnant Women in the US: NHANES 2003–2004," *Environmental Health Perspectives*, January 14, 2011, http://ehp03.niehs.nih.gov/article/info:doi/10.1289/ehp.1002727 (accessed March 10, 2011).

3. Jeffrey Norris, "Chemicals in Environment Deserve Study for Possible Role in Fat Gain, Says Byers Award Recipient," UCSF News, December 15, 2010, http://www.ucsf.edu/news/2010/12/6017/obesity-pesticides-pollutants-toxins-and-drugs-linked-studies-c-elegans (accessed March 10, 2011).

4. CureZone.com, "Celery Seed (Apium Graveolens), Celery Seed Tea," http://curezone.com/cleanse/kidney/Celery-seeds.asp (accessed March 10, 2011).

5. Mayo Clinic Staff, "Kidney Stones: Alternative Medicine," January 30, 2010, http://www.mayoclinic.com/health/kidney-stones/DS00282/DSECTION=alternative-medicine (accessed March 10, 2011).

6. University of Maryland Medical Center, "Complementary Medicine: Cranberry," November 17, 2008, http://www.umm.edu/altmed/articles/cranberry-000235.htm (accessed March 10, 2011).

7. Mehmet Oz and Mike Roizen, "Give Your Liver a Break: Avoid Toxins," *Wichita Eagle*, November 9, 2010, http://www.kansas.com/2010/11/09/1580014/give-your-liver-a-break-avoid.html#ixzz1CNfMO7Ov (accessed March 10, 2011).

8. Ibid.

9. Nina Walsh, naturopathic physician and detoxification expert, contributed this information from her lecture on the Health & Fitness Cruise. For more information on Dr. Nina Walsh, see Appendix A.

6—THE LIVING FOODS DIET PLAN

1. Laura Blue, "One Meal to Good (or Bad) Health," *Time*, January 15, 2008, http://www.time.com/time/health/article/0,8599,1703644,00.html (accessed March 6, 2011).

2. Virginia Worthington, "Nutritional Quality of Organic Versus Conventional Fruits, Vegetables, and Grains," *Journal of Alternative and Complementary Medicine* 7, no. 2 (2001): 161–173.

3. Switzer, "Bio-Photon Nutrition and Wild Green Energy Cocktails for Optimal Health (English)."

4. Garance Burke, "Methyl Iodide Approved for Use in California," HuffingtonPost.com, December 1, 2010, http://www.huffingtonpost.com/2010/12/01/methyl-iodide-approved-fo_n_790748.html (accessed March 11, 2011).

5. Joseph Mercola with Rachel Droege, "How Many Pesticides Are in Your Food? Find Out Now!", March 10, 2004, http://articles.mercola.com/sites/articles/archive/2004/03/10/pesticides-food.aspx (accessed March 9, 2011).

6. Maryland Pesticide Network, "Pesticide News," http://www.mdpestnet.org/resource/news/2010.htm (accessed February 7, 2010).

7. Vikki Katz, "Apples, Pears, and Pesticides—Protecting Children From Pesticide Residue," *Sierra*, September 2001, http://findarticles.com/p/articles/mi_m1525/is_5_86/ai_77279558/ (accessed March 22, 2011).

8. Melissa J. Perry and Frederick R. Bloom, "Perceptions of Pesticide-Associated Cancer Risks Among Farmers: A Qualitative Assessment," *Human Organization* 57 (1998): 342–349.

9. Maria Rodale "Organic Can Feed the World," *PCC Sound Consumer*, September 2010.

10. Ibid.

11. Jon Ungoed-Thomas, "Official: Organic Really Is Better," *Sunday Times*, October 28, 2007, http://www.timesonline.co.uk/tol/news/uk/health/article2753446.ece (accessed January 28, 2010).

12. Worthington, "Nutritional Quality of Organic Versus Conventional Fruits, Vegetables, and Grains"; US Department of Agriculture, *Pesticide Data Program: Annual Summary Calendar Year 2005* (Washington: Agricultural Marketing Service, 2006), http://www.ams.usda.gov/AMSv1.0/getfile?dDocName=STELPRDC5049946 (accessed February 3, 2011).

13. Fintan Dunne, "Organophosphates Implicated in Mad Cow Disease," http://www.laleva.cc/environment/insecticide_bse.html (accessed December 11, 2010).

14. J. D. Decuypere, "Radiation, Irradiation, and Our Food Supply," *The Decuypere Report*, http://www.healthalternatives2000.com/food-supply-report.html (accessed March 11, 2011).

15. Ibid.

16. Ibid.

17. US Food and Drug Administration, "Regulation of Foods Derived From Plants," statement of Lester M. Crawford before the Subcommittee on Conservation, Rural Development, and Research House Committee on Agriculture, June 17, 2003, http://www.fda.gov/NewsEvents/Testimony/ucm161037.htm (accessed March 11, 2011).

18. Mavis Butcher, "Genetically Modified Food—GM Foods List and Information," Disabled-World.com, September 22, 2009 http://www .disabled-world.com/fitness/gm-foods.php (accessed March 11, 2011).

19. Ibid.

20. Ronnie Cummins, "The Road Ahead: Steps Toward a Global Uprising," Organic Consumers Association, December 9, 2010, http://www .organicconsumers.org/articles/article_22174.cfm (accessed March 11, 2011).

21. G. C. Smith, "Dietary Supplementation of Vitamin E to Cattle to Improve Shelf Life and Case Life of Beef for Domestic and International Markets," Colorado State University, referenced in EatWild.com, "Summary of Important Health Benefits of Grassfed Meats, Eggs, and Dairy," http://www .eatwild.com/healthbenefits.htm (accessed March 11, 2011).

22. W. G. Kruggel, R. A. Field, G. J. Miller, K. M. Horton, and J. R. Busboom, "Influence of Sex and Diet on Lutein in Lamb Fat," *Journal of Animal Science* 54 (1982): 970–975.

23. World-wire.com, "American Public Health Association Supports Ban on Hormonal Milk and Meat," news release, November 13, 2009, http://www .world-wire.com/news/0911130001.html (accessed March 11, 2011).

24. ConsumerReports.org. "Chicken: Arsenic and Antibiotics," July 2007, http://www.consumerreports.org/cro/food/food-safety/animal-feed-and-food/animal-feed-and-the-food-supply-105/chicken-arsenic-and-antibiotics/index.htm (accessed March 11, 2011).

25. Tabitha Alterman, "Eggciting News!" MotherEarthNews.com, October 15, 2008, http://www.motherearthnews.com/Relish/Pastured-Eggs-Vitamin-D -Content.aspx (accessed March 11, 2011).

26. Ibid.

27. S. E. Swithers and T. L. Davidson, "A Role for Sweet Taste: Calorie Predictive Relations in Energy Regulation by Rats," *Behavioral Neuroscience* 122, no. 1 (February 2008): 161–173, referenced in ScienceDaily.com, "Artificial Sweeteners Linked to Weight Gain," February 11, 2008, http:// www .sciencedaily.com/releases/2008/02/080210183902.htm (accessed March 11, 2011).

28. L. Scalfi, A. Coltorti, and F. Contaldo, "Postprandial Thermogenesis in Lean and Obese Subjects After Meals Supplemented With Medium-Chain and Long-Chain Triglycerides," *American Journal of Clinical Nutrition* 53, no. 5 (May 1, 1991): 1130–1133.

29. Ogbolu, Oni, Daini, and Oloko, "*In Vitro* Antimicrobial Properties of Coconut Oil on Candida Species in Ibadan, Nigeria."

30. "Vegetable Oils/Fatty Acid Composition, Hexane Residues, Declaration, Pesticides (Organic Culinary Oils Only)," a joint campaign Basel city (specialist laboratory) and Basel county, http://www.kantonslabor-bs.ch/ files/berichte/Report0424.pdf (accessed March 11, 2011).

31. S. Couvreur, C. Hurtaud, C. Lopez, L. Delaby, and J. L. Peyraud, "The Linear Relationship Between the Proportion of Fresh Grass in the Cow Diet, Milk Fatty Acid Composition, and Butter Properties," *Journal of Dairy Science* 89, no. 6 (June 2006): 1956–1969, as referenced in EatWild. com, "Summary of Important Health Benefits of Grassfed Meats, Eggs, and Dairy."

32. Ibid.

33. S. O'Keefe, S. Gaskins-Wright, V. Wiley, and I-C. Chen, "Levels of Trans Geometrical Isomers of Essential Fatty Acids in Some Unhydrogenated U.S. Vegetable Oils," *Journal of Food Lipids* 1, no. 3 (September 1994): 165–176, referenced in WestonAPrice.org, "The Oiling of America," January 1, 2000, http://www.westonaprice.org/know-your-fats/525-the-oiling-of-america .html (accessed March 11, 2011).

34. *New York Times*, "Fat in Margarine Is Tied to Heart Problems," May 16, 1994, http://www.nytimes.com/1994/05/16/us/fat-in-margarine-is-tied-to -heart-problems.html (accessed March 11, 2011).

35. Alice Park, "Can Sugar Substitutes Make You Fat?" *Time*, February 10, 2008, http://www.time.com/time/health/article/0,8599,1711763,00.html (accessed March 11, 2011).

36. Woodrow C. Monte, "Aspartame: Methanol and Public Health," *Journal of Applied Nutrition* 36, no. 1 (1984): 44, referenced in documentary *Sweet Misery* (Tucson, AZ: Sound and Fury Productions, 2004), http://www .soundandfury.tv/pages/sweet%20misery.html (accessed March 11, 2011).

37. Ibid., also, Dani Veracity, "The Link Between Aspartame and Brain Tumors: What the FDA Never Told You About Artificial Sweeteners," NaturalNews .com, September 22, 2005, http://www.naturalnews.com/011804.html (accessed March 11, 2011).

38. Citizens for Health, "Chairman of Citizens for Health Declares FDA Should Review Approval of Splenda," press release, September 22, 2008, http:// www .globenewswire.com/newsroom/news.html?d=150785 (accessed March 11, 2011), referenced in Joanne Waldron, "Duke University Study Links Splenda to Weight Gain, Health Problems," NaturalNews.com, October 20, 2008, http://www.naturalnews.com/024543.html (accessed March 11, 2011).

39. Byron Richards, "High Fructose Corn Syrup Makes Your Brain Crave Food," 51commerce.net, April 1, 2009, http://www.51commerce.net/weight/ articles/high_fructose_corn_syrup_makes_your_brain_crave_food/index. htm (accessed March 11, 2011).

40. Yoshio Nagai et al., "The Role of Peroxisome Proliferator-Activated Receptor γ Coactivator-1 β in the Pathogenesis of Fructose-Induced Insulin Resistance," *Cell Metabolism* 9, no. 3 (March 4, 2009): 252–264.

7—The Living Revolution Menu Planner and Guide

1. Joseph Mercola, "Dr. Mercola's Comments: Chris Masterjohn—Criticism of *The China Study*, Part 1," January 8, 2011, http://articles.mercola.com/sites/ articles/archive/2011/01/08/chris-masterjohn-criticism-of-the-china-study .aspx (accessed March 11, 2011).

2. Joseph Mercola, "Criticism of *The China Study*: A Special Interview With Chris Masterjohn," transcript, http://mercola.fileburst.com/PDF/ ExpertInterviewTranscripts/InterviewChrisMasterjohnChinaStudy.pdf (accessed March 11, 2011).

3. Decuypere, "Radiation, Irradiation, and Our Food Supply."

4. Lita Lee, "Microwaves and Microwave Ovens," May 14, 2001, http://www .litalee.com/documents/Microwaves%20And%20Microwave%20Ovens.pdf (accessed March 14, 2011).

5. Decuypere, "Radiation, Irradiation, and Our Food Supply."

6. George J. Georgiou, "The Hidden Hazards of Microwave Cooking," *Journal for the American Association of Integrative Medicine* (online), April 2006, http://www.aaimedicine.com/jaaim/apr06/hazards.php (accessed March 14, 2011).

7. Anthony Wayne and Lawrence Newell, "The Hidden Hazards of Microwave Cooking," Health-Science.com, http://www.health-science.com/microwave_hazards.html (accessed March 14, 2011).

8—THE LIVING FOODS RECIPES

1. R. Akilen, A. Tsiami, D. Devendra, and N. Robinson, "Glycated Haemoglobin and Blood Pressure–Lowering Effect of Cinnamon in Multi-Ethnic Type 2 Diabetic Patients in the UK: A Randomized, Placebo-Controlled, Double-Blind Clinical Trial," *Diabetic Medicine* 27, no. 10 (October 2010): 1159–1167, http://onlinelibrary.wiley.com/doi/10.1111/j.1464-5491.2010.03079.x/full (accessed March 7, 2011).

2. Dae Jung Kim et al., "Magnesium Intake in Relation to Systemic Inflammation, Insulin Resistance, and the Incidence of Diabetes," *Diabetes Care* 33, no. 12 (December 2010): 2604–2610.

3. Sharon Barbour, "Cancer Boost From Whole Carrots," BBC News, June 16, 2009, http://news.bbc.co.uk/2/hi/health/8101403.stm (accessed March 7, 2011); Newcastle University Press Office, "Carrot Compound Reduces Cancer Risk," http://www.ncl.ac.uk/press.office/press.release/item/?ref=1107939821 (accessed March 7, 2011).

4. S. Oommen, R. J. Anto, G. Srinivas, and D. Karunagaran, "Allicin (From Garlic) Induces Caspase-Mediated Apoptosis in Cancer Cells," *Europe Journal of Pharmacology* 485 (February 6, 2004): 97–103.

5. Paul Bergner and Sharol Tilgner, "Gastrointestinal—Herbal Treatment for Ulcers," *Medical Herbalism* 3, no. 3: 1, 4–6, http://www.medherb.com/Therapeutics/Gastrointestinal_-_Herbal_treatment_for_ulcers.htm (accessed March 7, 2011).

6. Jed W. Fahey et al., "Sulforaphane Inhibits Extracellular, Intracellular, and Antibiotic-Resistant Strains of *Helicobacter Pylori* and Prevents Benzo[a]pyrene-Induced Stomach Tumors," *Proceedings of the National Academy of Sciences* 99, no. 11 (May 28, 2002): 7610–7615.

7. G. Bergsson et al., "In Vitro Killing of Candida Albicans by Fatty Acids and Monoglycerides," *Antimicrobial Agents and Chemotherapy* 45, no. 11 (November 2001): 3209–3212.

8. *Orlando Sentinel*, "Study: Pecans May Have Neurological Benefits," *Vital Signs* (blog), June 11, 2010, http://blogs.orlandosentinel.com/health/2010/06/11/study-pecans-may-have-neurological-benefits/ (accessed March 7, 2011).

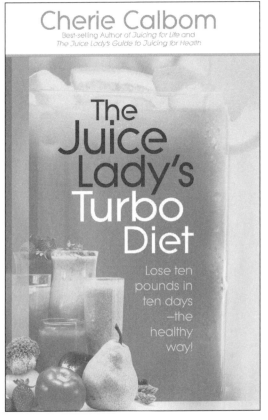

Lose ten pounds in ten days—
the healthy way!

Cherie Calbom serves up juicing tips, delicious recipies, and simple meal plans that will help you make juicing and raw foods an integral part of your weight-loss success.

Cherie Calbom
Best-selling Author of *Juicing for Life* and
The Juice Lady's Guide to Juicing for Health

The Juice Lady's Turbo Diet

Lose ten pounds in ten days —the healthy way!

978-1-61638-149-3 / $17.99

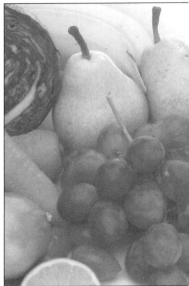

- Satisfy your bored taste buds.
- Cut your cravings.
- Detox your body.